Youth Offending in Transition

Youth offending – typified by images of young people roaming the streets in 'hoodies' – is an enduring preoccupation of media and government. But is this a true representation of young people's behaviour? How can we better understand the choices and constraints that young people face?

This book takes a new approach to youth crime by arguing that the transition from childhood to adulthood can be an isolating and disempowering experience for young people. Children and young people are inherently vulnerable because of their age and status – they are a minority group, with the potential for being exploited, discriminated against, dominated and disrespected by adults. *Youth Offending in Transition* explores how their treatment by adult society may lead young people to resort to crime as a means of gaining respect and kudos from their peers. Using concepts of capital and the narratives of young offenders themselves, this book is based on original research into the reasons why young people start and stop offending. It discusses the following topics:

* criminal theory and the significance of youth transitions to the 'age–crime curve';
* social identity and reputation amongst young people;
* social inequalities and their influence on youth transitions;
* the criminalization and discrimination of young people by adults;
* the importance of social recognition in reducing offending.

Youth Offending in Transition is an invaluable resource for students, academics and professionals working in criminology, youth justice, social policy, youth policy and social work.

Monica Barry is a Research Fellow at the University of Stirling, UK, working on youth offending, theories of desistance, youth transitions and social inclusion. She has a PhD in Criminology, is the Criminal Justice Research Advisor to the Association of Directors of Social Work in Scotland and recently edited *Youth Policy and Social Inclusion: Critical Debates with Young People,* published by Routledge in 2005.

Youth Offending in Transition

The search for social recognition

Monica Barry

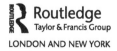

Routledge
Taylor & Francis Group

LONDON AND NEW YORK

First published 2006
by Routledge
2 Park Square, Milton Park, Abingdon, Oxon OX14 4RN

Simultaneously published in the USA and Canada
by Routledge
711 Third Ave, New York, NY 10017

Routledge is an imprint of the Taylor & Francis Group, an informa business

© 2006 Monica Barry

Typeset in Sabon by
HWA Text and Data Management, Tunbridge Wells

British Library Cataloguing in Publication Data
A catalogue record for this book is available from the British Library

Library of Congress Cataloging-in-Publication Data
A catalog record for this book has been requested

ISBN10: 0–415–36791–3 (hbk)
ISBN10: 0–415–36792–1 (pbk)
ISBN10: 0–203–02738–9 (ebk)

ISBN13: 978–0–415–36791–2 (hbk)
ISBN13: 978–0–415–36792–9 (pbk)
ISBN13: 978–0–203–02738–7 (ebk)

Dedicated to

Willy MacDonald

who hanged himself in prison, aged 17

His short life and accidental death epitomized everything that is currently known and yet to be understood about crime, criminality and criminal justice.

His life made me interested in working in this field.
His death made me committed to it.

Contents

Figures and tables

Figure

Tables

Acknowledgements

First and foremost, I want to thank the young people who took part in this study – although I am sure they won't thank me for mentioning their names! They gave up a lot of time and put in a lot of effort to make this study worthwhile. They not only offered me, as a complete stranger, warm hospitality in their own homes, but they also talked openly to me, and often with some difficulty, about their family backgrounds, their offending behaviour and their hopes for the future. My only wish is that this research will have a positive impact, if not on their own lives, then on the lives of their children.

This book is based on my PhD and is therefore a labour of love as much as a professional ambition. Thanks to my supervisors, Ian McIntosh and Gill McIvor, and my external examiners, Shadd Maruna and David Smith, for making it a constructive and positive (almost enjoyable!) experience.

My further thanks go to all my professional colleagues and personal friends who helped me to complete this study. Their help was highly valued and greatly appreciated in gaining access to the sample, formulating the research design, commenting constructively on endless drafts and supporting me with advice, encouragement, secretarial assistance, proof-reading and fine wine – all of which to varying degrees when I needed them most. These people are: Pat Allatt, Lorna Bell, Karen Bowler, Bill Burch, Terry Coppock, Joe Curran, John Dunlop, Ruth Emond, Roger Fuller, David Garland, Maureen Graham, Moyra Guilar, Graham Hamilton, David Hickling, Pam Lavery, Paul McFerran, Rhoda MacRae, Margaret Malloch, Richard Mitchell, Elizabeth Morrison, Ginny Morrow, Ronan O'Carroll, Helen Scott, Sue Warner and Susan Wiltshire.

Those that cannot be named, so as to ensure the confidentiality of the young people, are the staff of various institutions who facilitated my access to the young people, in particular the voluntary organization that worked most closely with the majority of respondents.

Finally, I would very much like to thank my husband, Roger Sidaway, and my family for being so patient, supportive (both academically and emotionally) and loving over the years that it has taken me to get my act together over this piece of work. The research meant nothing to them other than it meant a lot to me, and I greatly appreciated them being there.

Chapter 1

Introduction

The desire for recognition ... has no material object but seeks only a just evaluation of one's worth on the part of another human consciousness.

(Fukuyama, 1995: 358)

I just done it to be part of everybody.

(Janet, 21)

The desire for recognition

Whilst Fukuyama may not have quite the same way with words as Janet, they are in effect saying the same thing. Janet's recourse to offending in childhood was a pragmatic means of gaining recognition from her peers at a time when she had few other opportunities for integration and identity within the wider society. Moving through the phases of transition – from childhood, through youth to adulthood – can be an isolating and disempowering experience for young people, not least when they also lack political and economic power. Children and young people are thus inherently vulnerable because of their age and status and are, in effect, a minority group with the same potential for exploitation, discrimination, domination, disrespect and non-recognition by adults. It is little wonder, therefore, that they find solace in their peers in the transition to adulthood. This book demonstrates how important the peer group is to young people in transition. It also demonstrates how readily some young people may resort to crime as one means of gaining a valued reputation with others of similar age or status.

Whilst the discipline of criminology has recognized the importance of age in understanding offending, it has not fully grasped the significance of youth transitions to the 'age-crime curve'.[1] Whilst there are some notable examples of a developing interest in youth transitions within criminological circles (for example, Bottoms *et al.*, 2004; Sampson and Laub, 1993; Webster *et al.*, 2004), none has specifically tied the phases of transition with those of offending. The study on which this book is based draws on a combination of criminological theories, youth transitions theories and concepts of capital (power), and argues that youth transitions are influenced by age-related power imbalances, as is offending behaviour. The book investigates the possible linkages between the three phases of offending – onset, maintenance and desistance; and those of youth transitions – childhood, youth and adulthood. It is argued that the phases of offending run similar courses to the phases of youth transition and that offending in the transition to adulthood is one means of gaining status or capital during that transitionary period.

This book encapsulates the experiences and views of young people in transition who have been embroiled in the criminal justice system for prolonged periods in childhood and youth. Based on their views and through the use of the concept of capital developed by Pierre Bourdieu, this book develops the notion of 'social recognition' – namely, the attainment of a durable and legitimate combination of capital accumulation and expenditure – which may help us to understand why young people do or do not successfully desist from crime during the transition to adulthood. This is a novel formulation although it draws on earlier thinking about reputation and identity. Bromley (1993: 33), for example, suggests that disempowered individuals and groups are likely to focus on their immediate group for the development of identity and reputation: 'Membership of a minority group of like-minded individuals can be an effective buffer against a hostile majority'. Emler (1990) suggests that for young people with no other status or power, a bad reputation is often preferable to no reputation at all, since it at least gains one attention. He also suggests that law-abiding behaviour only offers one a reputation by default, whereas deviance has a more profound and immediate effect on one's reputation.

Given that young people are in a transitional phase in their lives, because of their age and status, and see themselves as increasingly dependent on friends as a 'buffer' between leaving childhood and attaining adulthood, then it is likely that reputations with peers will be deliberately and rapidly cultivated and may often not be sustainable. As will be seen from the findings of the research discussed in this book, many young people experience just such a lack of sustainability of reputations in youth, and many consciously discard such reputations in favour of more durable reputations in adulthood. Thus, modifications to their social identities are often made following a weakening of effective reputations in childhood and early youth, exacerbated by external constraints such as the criminal justice system:

> If people wish to break free from a particular social identity, they need to break free from the constraints of social circumstances, and the influence of particular people... conversely, if people want a particular sort of social identity, they need to submit to social constraints and influence.
>
> (Bromley, 1993: 57)

> I've still got a reputation as someone that I used to be, you know, that you remember, but people know now I've settled down with kids and keep my head down... Like I remember one of the boys seen me going to work dressed like this [in a suit] and they thought I was actually going to court! But that's because of the area that we live in.
>
> (Harry, 26)

This book tells young people's stories of that journey to break free from one particular social identity and to adopt another.

The criminalization of children and young people

Young people adopt diverse pathways in the transition to adulthood but are equally constrained by external factors, notably their minimal legal status and their restricted opportunities for meaningful further education and employment. The importance of social inequalities and social institutions in determining or undermining youth transitions is becoming increasingly apparent. Many young people are excluded from higher education (through a lack of qualifications or financial support), from employment opportunities and from housing. Nevertheless, the fact is that the majority of young people who are marginalized or otherwise disadvantaged within the labour market as elsewhere do not rebel against their predicament. On the contrary:

> The response of the unemployed to the aggravation of labour
> market disadvantage lies not in the development of some
> highly distinctive subculture, but in the reinforcement of more
> conventional working-class beliefs.
>
> (Gallie, 1994: 756, quoted in MacDonald, 1997: 175)

Conventionality, and young people's aspirations towards mainstream goals, are factors often ignored by both academics and policy makers in attempting to understand deviant behaviour in youth. There is also a growing body of evidence that young people are on the whole conformist and that their problems in youth are exacerbated by the pessimistic image and limited understanding that many adults have of them. Matza (1964: 27) has criticized positivist criminology for ignoring 'mundane and commonplace childhood activity' amongst children and young people, but there is also strong evidence from studies of offending behaviour more generally that crime is ubiquitous amongst all social classes and all ages.

Although the number of young people 'officially' involved in crime is minimal compared with the youth population as a whole, the political emphasis on youth crime has been exacerbated by media coverage which has highlighted the apparently spiralling 'problem' of children and young people. And yet when one ranks crimes in order of seriousness, one could arguably put street crime, prostitution and theft at the bottom of the hierarchy, and terrorism, business fraud and drug smuggling at the top. Indeed, offending by young people tends to be small-time and generally unsuccessful, but still gains a disproportionate level of attention from the media, the police and the criminal justice system. Whilst the number of children and young people in the population has decreased during the late twentieth century (and is not projected to rise over the following two decades at least) and whilst some 97 per cent of crimes go undetected in the UK, the criminal justice system is nevertheless costing the government over £16 billion a year, with much of that money going on 'chasing and punishing... adolescents armed with nothing more sophisticated than the sawn-off top of a Pepsi bottle' (Davies, 2003a: 1).

The legal status of children and young people as well as their image in the media changed from being considered victims and in need of protection in the early 1990s to unruly villains from whom the community needs to be protected in the late 1990s (Franklin, 2002). Many authors suggest that this shift was prompted by the murder of two-year-old James Bulger, whose death at the hands of two ten-year-old boys in 1993 seemed to totally undermine the concept of childhood as being a time of innocence, and of children as being 'cute and contented' (Franklin, 2002: 18). As Brown (1998: 2) suggests: 'The real violence of the Bulger case is arguably the violence it did to adult notions of childhood': social expectations are that whilst 'young people' may offend, 'children' should not. And yet the opposing notions of childhood as innocence versus childhood as deviance are not new, having appeared in literature since the time of the Enlightenment (Franklin, 2002). Nevertheless, children and young people generally are becoming the benchmark of anticipated behaviour over the whole of the life course, and as Cohen and Ainley (2000: 89) point out: 'young people have had to carry a peculiar burden of representation; everything they do, say, think or feel is scrutinized by an army of professional commentators for signs of the times'.

Since the mid-nineteenth century, social control mechanisms in relation to crime have focused predominantly on children and young people. However, towards the end of the twentieth century, such social control mechanisms had begun to *anticipate* rather than *react to* criminal behaviour through a broadening of the definition of crime to include the *potential* for crime. The Anti-Social Behaviour Bill (2003) gave the police the right to disperse groups of young people on the streets and to remove into care those deemed in need of greater control than that offered by their own families. Parenting orders, anti-social behaviour orders, curfews and electronic monitoring of children and young people have equally undermined their rights and those of their parents to freedom of expression and privacy (Brown, 1998). Brown argues that there is 'a recurring and ongoing preoccupation with the perceived threat to social stability posed by unregulated, undisciplined and disorderly youth outside adult control' (1998: 77).

This increasing scapegoating of children and young people as 'disorderly' masks the fact that over a third of children in the UK live in poverty (Franklin, 2002). In the 1980s and 1990s, social inequalities and class polarization became increasingly apparent and absolute poverty increased within a climate of reduced welfare provision and economic instability (Callinicos, 1999). According to some sociologists, this has resulted in increasing insecurity and risk, not least for children and young people in the transition to adulthood (Beck, 1992; Coles, 1995). It is suggested in the following chapters of this book that whilst longer-term opportunities for capital may be lacking for some young people in transition, offending can be used as a strategy, however temporary or misguided, to give them a valuable source of identity, status and recognition in an otherwise potentially marginalizing period in their lives. In this respect, the temporary nature of youth transitions and the lack of legitimate, longer-term capital during that transitional period are important factors in better understanding how, when and why offending and desistance occur.

Social recognition: a new perspective on youth transitions

Pierre Bourdieu's theory of social practice (1986), and in particular his concepts of social, economic, cultural and symbolic capital, are helpful in examining the imbalances in opportunities and status for young people in transition. His conceptual framework, described further in Chapter 3, was chosen specifically because it is a dynamic model that gives prominence and credence to the structural influences of time, space, status and class. Looking at the evidence from young people through the lens of Bourdieu's concept of capital, it seems that the desire for capital through integration and status is an important factor both in the transition to adulthood and in the process of offending and desistance. The concept of capital cuts across the boundaries between childhood, youth and adulthood, but the lack of sustainability and legitimacy of such capital in transition makes recourse to offending more likely. Because of their transitional situation, many young people lack the status and opportunities for full citizenship. They thus have limited capacity for what I term 'social recognition': the attainment of a combination of accumulation and expenditure of capital that is both durable and legitimate. The concept of 'social recognition' is used to better explain the sequence of events and thinking surrounding young people's offending over time and to combine both agency and structure in the transition to adulthood and desistance.

In linking the phases of offending with the phases of transition, it is possible to engage with the temporary nature of youth offending and to draw comparisons between changes in offending over time and the contrasting levels of capital accumulated in the transition to adulthood. There is a seeming convergence of the two pathways of offending and youth transitions, and the accounts by young people of their offending over time strongly suggest that such behaviour is a personal means (capital accumulation) to a social end (capital expenditure). The pathways of offending and youth transitions suggest both movement in time and individual agency and, as such, support the argument in this book that offending is a transient occupation, its duration dependent not only on external structural factors but also on individual self-determination. Because of their relative powerlessness in youth, certain young people lack the opportunities to spend as well as accumulate legitimate and durable capital. Whilst offending enables the accumulation of capital in the short term, it does not enable the accumulation or expenditure of capital in the longer term. It is suggested that desistance comes not with age *per se* in the transition to adulthood but with increased opportunities for social recognition through, for example, generativity[2] and responsibility taking. This central argument of the book is explored in greater detail in Chapter 7.

The young people in this book

The narratives reported in this book are from a study of young people that I undertook in Scotland in 2000–1, which set out to explore their perceptions of why they start offending, continue offending over a period of time and stop offending, whether there were gender differences emerging from this analysis, and whether there was a common thread between their reasons for starting, continuing and stopping offending (for a broader discussion of the methodology, see Appendix A). The 40 respondents – 20 young men and 20 young women – all came from socio-economic backgrounds that restricted their opportunities for stable employment, adequate housing and social identity. The sample is unusual in that it comprises 40 young people who had been heavily involved in offending in the past but also includes a combination of persisters and desisters as well as an equal gender mix. Compared to many other studies of offending and desistance, this sample consisted entirely of young people who had been high-tariff, serious offenders for a substantial part of their offending lives. Four-fifths of the young people started offending as 'children' (i.e. at the age of 15 or under), their reasons being mainly because of a lack of attention or love, to seek encouragement or recognition, to earn money or as a (latent) reaction to (past) traumas in their lives. Many came from families marred by death, illness, separation and transience, and many felt unloved or uncared for as a result. Indeed, the school setting may have offered these young people respite from marginalization or familial neglect or abuse and gave them an opportunity to create a social identity for themselves. This book gives this group of young people an opportunity to describe and explain how and why they became involved in crime, and will hopefully go some way towards developing a greater understanding of youth offending more generally. Throughout the book, quotations by the young people in the sample which are used to illustrate points made in the text are referenced by a pseudonym followed by the age of the respondent at interview – for example: 'Anna, 21'.

Working with 'wobbly constructs'

Crime has been described as a 'wobbly construct' (Heidensohn, 1985), lacking a clear definition, which makes the interpretation of behaviour that results in crime an equally dubious activity. Gottfredson and Hirschi (1990) argue that criminology's position of trying to understand criminality generally is flawed if it cannot first adopt a universal concept of 'crime'. Various sets of literature define crime in different ways, for example: 'an action defined by the law... which, if detected, will lead to some kind of sanction being employed against the perpetrator' (Emsley, 1994: 150); and 'banned or controlled behaviour which is likely to attract punishment or disapproval' (Downes and Rock, 1988: 28). In this book, the terms 'offending' or 'offending behaviour' are taken to mean acts or behaviour which, whether or not detected, warrant *potential* legal proceedings being taken against the individual.

As with the notion of crime, the term '*persistence*' proves difficult to define clearly. Various authors describe persistence in various ways, depending on either official reconviction data or on self-report data. Jamieson *et al.* (1999) define self-reported persistence as pertaining to those who say they have committed at least one serious or several less serious offences in the previous 12 months, and these authors also use persistence to differentiate that group from 'resisters' and 'desisters'. Farrington (1995) suggests that a 'chronic' persistent label can only be placed on those individuals with six previous convictions by the age of 18. Muncie (1999: 308) avoids being specific by suggesting that persistence means 'the recurring notion that a small group of offenders make up a disproportionate part of the "crime problem"'. Given the likely variations between self-reported and official data, disparities in police practice according to the age and gender of alleged offenders, and changes in offending over time, the term 'persistence' is naturally problematic. In this book, persistence relates to those who have been convicted of at least three offences at the time of interview (although the young men had a minimum of 14 such offences – see Appendix B).

However, persistence not only relates to the level of offending (as measured by the numbers of convictions) but also to the frequency of offending. Throughout the book, I have departed from usual practice in choosing to replace persistence with the word 'maintenance', since persistence often suggests not only dogged obstinacy or purposefulness, but also increased frequency of offending. Maintenance, on the other hand, suggests the possibility of merely keeping going, with or without purpose, and can denote a reduction as well as an increase in offending behaviour over time.

Desistance likewise varies in definition, from 'the voluntary termination of serious criminal participation' (Shover, 1996: 121) to 'the maintenance of crime-free behaviour... the study of *continuity* rather than change' (Maruna, 2001: 26–7, emphasis in original). This latter definition highlights the concept of desistance as *process* (narrative data) rather than *outcome* (reconviction data). Desistance as outcome infers a complete cessation of all offending behaviour but is problematic in not allowing for the 'hidden' incidence of criminal behaviour which, whilst illegal, is not labelled if not detected. Various studies classify desisters as those who have been offence-free for a twelve-month period, although one study suggests a timescale of eleven years for desistance to have occurred (Farrington and Hawkins, 1991). Within this study, desistance was defined purely by the respondents themselves, although it was possible to corroborate their perceptions and timescales with official Scottish Criminal Record Office (SCRO) data on reconviction rates.

I have in this book also adopted the expression '*offending phase*', rather than 'career' or 'trajectory', as a means of including agency or self-determination, dynamics, flexibility and the notion of temporary rather than more permanent change. To Coles (1995), 'career' means 'the sequence of statuses through which young people pass [which] sets in train a series of social processes which has the potentiality to "determine" the likely course of a young person's future status sequence' (ibid.: 8). He does not suggest an automatic progression (or digression) from one sequence to another, but states that each sequence has the capacity to inform future sequencing.

The word 'trajectory', on the other hand, suggests more of an automatic progression (or digression) from one sequence to another: 'the connotation of young people being somehow propelled along awaiting channels towards predetermined destinations' (Bates and Riseborough, 1993, quoted in Coles, 1995: 12).

The term '*young people*' is used extensively by criminologists and other academics in research, policy and legal documents worldwide, although arguably without strict definition. In the UK, for example, 'young people' tends to refer to those between the ages of 15 and 25 (Jones, 1995), in Australia those between the ages of 13 and 25 (Cunneen and White, 2002) and in Finland those up to the age of 29 within the Youth Work Act (2002) at least (Tammi, 2004, pers. comm.). The people described in this book are collectively referred to as 'young people', although they range in age from 18 to 30.[3] However, by including those in their late twenties, the research covers the upper age by which desistance is usually said to have occurred for most offenders (Blumstein *et al.*, 1988).

The layout of this book

This chapter has described the context of the book, current understandings of youth criminality and criminalization and relevant concepts that will be drawn upon in the course of the book. Chapter 2, while not attempting to provide a literature review, examines some of the issues arising from criminological theories relating to offending and desistance which are deemed to be of pertinence to the book's overall aims. Chapter 3 examines a wider set of theoretical literature pertaining to youth transitions which is deemed crucial in informing a greater understanding of the prevalence of offending amongst young people. It thus fills a gap in criminology, by placing offending in a wider social context of youth transitions. The chapter also includes a brief résumé of Pierre Bourdieu's theory of practice (1977; 1986), and describes his concepts of capital and their relevance to offending and desistance in transition. Chapters 4, 5 and 6 focus on the views and experiences of the young people about, respectively, starting, continuing and stopping offending, interspersing their narratives with comparators from the literature described in earlier chapters. These three chapters utilize broadly similar parameters in presenting the data: what factors influenced the young people's propensity or otherwise to offend and the advantages and disadvantages of starting, continuing and stopping offending. They also highlight particular stories through the use of case studies.

Chapter 7 progresses the analysis of Bourdieu's concepts of capital in relation to offending, desistance and youth transitions, developing the notion of capital expenditure as well as accumulation. Again it draws on case study material to illustrate these young people's capacity and opportunities to spend their capital through conventional means, namely, responsibility taking and generativity, thereby increasing the likelihood of desistance through 'social recognition'. Finally, Chapter 8 draws together the key points from the book and highlights the importance of Bourdieu's concepts of capital in better understanding youth offending in transition. There are also suggestions made in relation to the considerable scope for further research on social recognition, a concept which has the potential to provide a lasting alternative to offending for young people, both in theory and practice.

Chapter 2

Offending and desistance in theory

> ... in so far as youth raises its voice at all, the cry is for jobs, for incorporation; their concern is not to subvert a social order but to join it.
>
> (Mungham, 1982: 38)

Introduction

As mentioned in Chapter 1, conventionality amongst young people is often ignored when attempting to come to terms with deviant behaviour in youth (MacDonald, 1997). Indeed, academics, policy makers and the media tend to give disproportionate attention to young people's criminal activity, thus sensationalizing the 'problem'. Policy interest in what works with offenders has often undermined an exploration of issues relating to how and why certain interventions work (Maruna, 1998), how and why indirect interventions may impact on offending behaviour (e.g. poverty, social networks and employment or educational opportunities) and what offenders themselves think are the problems. Whilst youth justice *research* in particular has been invaluable in raising our academic awareness of the issues surrounding offending amongst young people, it has not always impacted positively on the direction in which youth justice *policy* is heading. There are anomalies in our understanding of what constitutes offending behaviour between and within cultures and how that behaviour should be defined and measured. There is also confusion about causes versus correlates of offending. Causes suggest that a negation of offending behaviour would come about from an absence of those factors directly influencing the behaviour. Correlates, on the other hand, suggest only potential association, and thus are unable to separate out cause and effect. However, rarely do policy makers address the causes so much as tinker with the correlates of crime. This chapter briefly explores the literature since the 1950s on why young people might start offending and the now burgeoning literature on why the majority of young people stop offending. It is not a definitive review of the criminological literature but an illustration of the challenges for current policy and the potential for further research.[1]

Theories of offending in youth

According to much criminological literature, young people offend for one or more of the following reasons: because of their age; through rational choice for utilitarian, monetary or hedonistic gain; because of an inability to achieve one's aspirations conventionally within mainstream society; as a result of a lack of self-control; because of the influence of others; in pursuit of excitement and cultural innovation; or because of a lack of socialization. A further school of thought suggests that offending behaviour is ubiquitous and normal but that it may be socially or politically labelled as a problem so as to justify or ensure social control.

Many of the criminological theories since the mid-twentieth century or so have focused on people's blocked aspirations towards mainstream values and goals (e.g. strain theory). These blockages may arise because of inherent traits in individuals resulting from bio-social deficits in childhood, such as low self-control, inadequate socialization or overly-hedonistic values. They may also arise because of 'misguided' moral reasoning (e.g. social control or rational choice theories), because of one's status in the social hierarchy (e.g. subcultural theories) or because of a lack of status and employment in adulthood (e.g. social bonds). More recent radical theories of crime have also suggested that the labelling of individuals or certain youth cultures as 'criminal' may lead to an escalation of crime or marginalization (e.g. labelling theory and cultural criminology), and that relative poverty and inequality within communities may result in differential access to limited opportunities (e.g. left realism). In relation to young people, the lack of adequate parenting or socialization as children, the influence of peers, the vagaries of the labour market or a delayed transition to adulthood may result in a tendency to 'drift' between mainstream conventionality and subcultural delinquency (Matza, 1964).

However, the literature on onset of offending is sparse in its coverage of certain key issues. First, the criminological literature to date has been unable to accommodate temporal, cultural and social changes which impact on offending behaviour. Subcultural theory (Cloward and Ohlin, 1961; Miller, 1958), for example, may have been a likely explanation for the prevalent gang mentality of the 1950s and 60s in the USA, especially amongst black Americans (MacDonald, 1997), but was not found to translate easily into a British context (Downes, 1966). Equally, Matza (1964; 1969) placed a lot of blame at the door of sociological positivism for imagining a subcultural milieu that ties adolescents to a seemingly timeless commitment to deviant behaviour and anti-conventional beliefs. He questioned how subcultural theory allowed for the fact that such a commitment to crime would be suddenly set aside when the young person matured, a common criticism with many theories of criminality. Similarly, as with subcultural theory, cultural criminologists (Fenwick and Hayward, 2000; Ferrell and Sanders, 1995) highlight the 'group' and focus on spectacular cultural activities amongst young people, whereas much youthful offending is often an individual phenomenon and is neither culturally-specific nor 'spectacular' enough to attract the attention of the media. Hebdige (1979: 122, quoted in Wyn and White, 1997: 83) has suggested that youth culture can either be 'a major dimension' or 'a slight distraction' in young people's lives, depending amongst other things on their need for escapism or integration. Much youth culture requires little commitment, is not labelled as problematic, and is therefore not criminalized. Watching a licensed television is a case in point.

Second, few theories of crime to date are applicable to women's offending or to the fact that law enforcement is predominantly a male preserve. Female offending has largely been ignored because of its usually low-profile and infrequent nature. Conviction data highlight a marked gender ratio between the sexes, and Heidensohn (1985) suggests that this prompted an examination by feminists since the 1970s of why women tend to conform rather than to offend: 'the most striking thing about female behaviour… is how notably conformist to social mores women are' (ibid.: 11). Yet, the fact that women commit fewer crimes than men, that such crimes are less serious, and that women are less likely to be victimized, has had little impact on criminological thought until recently. Women's offending differs significantly from men's in frequency and it is a myth to suggest that women offenders are mainly involved in shoplifting and prostitution as a result of poverty or economic marginality (Brown, 1998; Heidensohn, 1994; Morris, 1987). An analysis of why women offend less, why their offending rate is rising faster than men's for certain offences and why the law treats them differently, could arguably enable a greater understanding of not only women's offending but that of men as well (Heidensohn, 1985; 1994).

Third, many theories of offending cannot readily explain changes in rates, seriousness and frequency, nor can they explain why many offenders do *not* – as well as do – stop offending in adulthood. Offenders are as likely to be influenced by significant others and events in deciding to *continue* offending as they are in deciding whether and when to stop offending, as is argued in differential association theory (Sutherland and Cressey, 1970). Likewise, right realism (Wilson, 1975) and rational choice theory (Cornish and Clarke, 1986) cannot account for the often futile and mismanaged behaviour of many law breakers (Burnett, 2003; Rutter *et al.*, 1998; Shover, 1996) who continue to pursue criminal careers against all the odds. Equally, strain theory (Agnew, 1992; Cohen, 1955; Greenberg, 1979; Merton, 1957) cannot easily account for middle class delinquency nor for the intermittent nature of some offending or indeed the sudden and inexplicable cessation of offending altogether.

Fourth, developmental perspectives (Matsueda and Heimer, 1997; Moffitt, 1993; Thornberry, 1997) have possibly deflected attention away from the social and political construction of age and youth transitions. Whilst the individual implications of age *per se* are important in understanding offending, there are external, power-related and political implications of youth transitions (such as human rights, citizenship and age-related structural constraints) which have largely been ignored in criminological research. For example, a focus on the need for young people to find work or merely to become 'employable' in order to reduce their offending overshadows the need to reassess the discriminatory nature of an adult-oriented labour market.

Finally, the theories which address young people's propensity to start offending are rarely compatible with those which address their propensity to stop offending, and yet one might expect a certain continuity or logical progression from onset through to desistance. For example, certain theories of offending argue that young people are disaffected by or rebel against middle class values and opportunities, and yet they are nevertheless often found to stop offending without ever having gained such values or opportunities. This book thus argues for a more combined approach to criminological theory which purposefully addresses the issues that are common to both starting and stopping offending.

Theories of desistance

Until the 1980s, there had been few theoretical explanations offered within criminology for desistance (Glaser, 1980), although there is currently increasing interest in this aspect of the discipline (e.g. Farrall, 2000; 2002; Graham and Bowling, 1995; Jamieson *et al.*, 1999; Leibrich, 1993; Maruna, 2001; Sampson and Laub, 1993; Shover and Thompson, 1992). As with the commonalities in the literature on offending, those relating to desistance are broadly similar in range, stressing what are seen to be the achievement of individual aspirations towards generally available mainstream goals. The literature on desistance has also focused predominantly on changed values and perceptions of risk (issues of agency) or on increased opportunities for conventional living (issues of structure), but rarely in tandem. However, whilst the desistance literature is now increasingly seeking the views of offenders and ex-offenders themselves, thus combining micro-level structural factors (such as access to employment or family relationships) with individual narratives, such literature still tends to avoid the need to address the macro-level structural constraints and imbalances within society (poverty, responsibility, human rights) and the socio-legal impact of transitions on young people's lived experience of youth.

Theories which combine agency and structure (see, for example, Farrall and Bowling, 1999), recognize the limitations of approaches that single out personality factors or structural factors alone. What is also increasingly recognized by academics in the field is the need to embed such theories in the narratives of offenders themselves. Maruna (2001) acknowledges that social factors and age, for example, are positively correlated with desistance, but points out that offenders' narratives are equally important and can supplement other explanations of crime. He thus stresses the role of narrative theory – using personal autobiographies in social enquiry – as both a methodological tool and a theoretical framework and within the desistance literature it incorporates aspects of human behaviour and perception not necessarily covered by maturational or social control theories. Maruna (2001) suggests that little empirical research has explored the changes in individuals' subjective perceptions between the processes of persistence and desistance.

Farrall and Bowling (1999) draw on structuration theory (Giddens, 1984) and life-course perspectives (Sampson and Laub, 1993) to propose a developmental theory of desistance using offenders' own narratives. Deploying the work of Giddens in criminology is a relatively new phenomenon (Bottoms and Wiles, 1992; Farrall and Bowling, 1999), but Farrall and Bowling have shown that the concepts of duality of structure, power, social identities and position-practices are useful empirical tools in exploring young people's experiences of desistance. Farrall and Bowling's contention is that power differentials *within* individuals over the life course will influence the 'timing and pace' of desistance (1999: 265). Within their qualitative sample, these authors found that positive changes in roles and responsibilities within one's family or immediate social network could create an equally positive change in one's attitude to offending. Like Farrall and Bowling, Leibrich (1993) also found that people reduced their offending behaviour through revised personal values, having something of value in life (material or social), developing self-respect and settling down. However, she also suggests that offending may have started because of financial or social deprivation: 'People who have nothing of value have nothing to lose. People who have no sense of belonging have no social status to risk' (ibid.: 240).

Several key issues are mentioned here that have proved problematic for academics in the desistance field. First, desistance is not an easily measurable phenomenon because of the difficulty of identifying *when* desistance has occurred and authors use a range of methods of data collection and differing lengths of time in measuring periods of non-offending. Desistance is often said not to be conclusive evidence of stopped offending until 7–10 years of an offence-free lifestyle (Farrington, 1986): relapses are common and the path to desistance crooked (Leibrich, 1993).

Second, relatively few studies have looked at desistance from a gendered perspective or included the first-hand experiences of female offenders. Although Jamieson *et al.* (1999) suggest that females report similar types of offending as their male counterparts, they also suggest that young women find it easier to desist from offending than young men. Graham and Bowling (1995) argue that whilst young women do indeed grow out of crime for whatever reason, some young men actually grow into it. Whilst they found young women to be more successful at making the transition from childhood to adulthood on leaving school (in terms of leaving home, forming stable relationships and becoming more economically and socially independent), young men are less likely to successfully make that transition until well into their twenties, partly because of greater peer pressure for the men in their sample.

Finally, studies of desistance have not readily differentiated between what has been termed 'life-course persistent' and 'adolescent-limited' offending (Moffitt, 1993), given that there may be a diverse range of factors differentiating the two types of offender. Sampson and Laub (1993) suggest that the maturational reform approach to offending (Glueck and Glueck, 1940) has focused on adolescents in a vacuum, divorced from their origins as children and from their ultimate destination as adults. Thus, they stress the need for a life-course perspective. However, as implied above, age is a confounding variable and needs to be analysed within a wider social, political and economic context. For example, it could be argued that with age comes a greater awareness of risk factors as well as the concomitant fear of having something to lose by offending, although as Leibrich (1993) points out, unless one has something of value in the first place, one is unlikely to be aware of having something to lose.

Offending and desistance in parallel

The criminological literature on offending and desistance can suggest no common thread that enables an understanding of offending and desistance as parts of the same process. On the one hand, the literature on onset of offending focuses on self-control, social control and opportunities that meet young people's expectations for personal identity and social development. However, such theories tend not to relate offending to the socio-legal position of many disadvantaged young people in the transition to adulthood, nor can they readily explain differences between ethnicity, gender, class and age, and variations in rates and types of offending over time.

On the other hand, the literature on desistance focuses predominantly on 'trigger points' during the life course which are likely to encourage desistance, but cannot account for desistance where no such trigger points exist. Whilst many young offenders, notably those from working class backgrounds, may not have opportunities such as stable employment, a home and family of their own or access to supportive mechanisms of informal social control (Sampson and Laub, 1993), nevertheless, the majority of such young people still stop offending. Sampson and Laub (1993) stress the importance of social ties but even that concept has not proved empirically rigorous. Social ties such as employment, school achievement, marriage and parenthood have not always been shown to be associated with a reduction in offending (Sampson and Laub, 1993; Leibrich, 1993; Rutter, 1996). As with the literature on offending, much of the literature on desistance views the cessation of offending as occurring in a vacuum, ignoring the possibility of offending as a process of change over time and space. Nevertheless, some of the theorists of onset of offending have potential commonalities with desistance. In particular, Gottfredson and Hirschi's theory of self-control offers the potential to explain both onset and desistance, as does rational choice theory and Matza's theory of drift. However, desistance in these theories is seen more as a negation or absence of the original problems that caused offending to start, rather than being seen as a proactive process of change in itself. In addition, these particular theories are not strong in explaining how that change might take place, only that it may.

Because theories of offending and desistance cannot adequately differentiate over time between the three phases of onset, maintenance and desistance, there is little continuity between such theories. Indeed, two particular studies of offending and desistance (Blumstein *et al.*, 1988; Leibrich, 1993) have gone so far as to suggest that the correlates associated with starting offending need not match or correspond with those associated with stopping offending:

> Theories regarding the causes of crime will very likely have to distinguish the factors stimulating individuals to become involved in crime from the factors ... inhibiting termination of criminal careers ... In the criminal career approach, by contrast, the different criminal career features can each have different correlates and predictors and they are not necessarily interrelated.
>
> (Blumstein *et al.*, 1988: 4–5)

> Assumptions about why and how people go straight tend to be based on the related but not necessarily pertinent question of why and how they get into trouble
>
> (Leibrich, 1993: 17)

Such a diagnosis of the problem, which basically sees onset and desistance as two discrete topics of academic interest, is perhaps unhelpful in understanding offending and desistance as a *process* of change for the individual. What is also problematic about much of the criminological literature on both onset and desistance is the lack of clarity about what is an individually-derived versus an externally-determined explanation for offending behaviour, an extension of the controversy over structure versus agency. As an example, in relation to theories of onset, strain theory generally suggests that the individual is somehow propelled into a criminal role based on an incapacity to fulfil personal aspirations because of external constraints. This theory comes under the rubric of sociological positivism, where heterogeneity and choice are underplayed in favour of consensus and determinism. As Muncie (1999: 112) suggests in relation to positivistic criminological theory: '... people are propelled into crime by circumstances over which they have no control... crime is *caused* either by individual "pathologies" and/or by precipitative social and economic conditions' (emphasis in original). If one asks individuals involved in crime whether, on the one hand, they are propelled reluctantly into a life of crime or, on the other hand, choose to have aspirations which crime can further meantime, their responses may be ambiguous or contradictory. They may at some times play down their own control of the situation and at other times blame only themselves (Maruna, 2001; Matza, 1964). Such behaviour is, nevertheless, often based on quite rational calculation: the individual chooses to behave in a certain way – albeit within the confines of external constraints. Therefore, structural versus individual explanations of crime are not mutually exclusive but highlight both the complementary and dichotomous relationships between structure and agency.

One criminological theory in particular goes some way towards bridging that gap between structure and agency and offending and desistance, and is worthy of some expansion at this point. Matza's theory of drift (1964) suggests that young people are not compelled (by their environment) nor coerced (by learnt or encouraged behaviour) to offend, but drift in and out of deviant behaviour over a temporary and transient period during adolescence. Matza points out that the majority of people are conformist in behaviour and attitude and young people are generally no different in their beliefs and values than their counterparts in the wider society. This at least partial conformity to law-abiding behaviour is evidenced by offenders' frequent demonstrations of guilt or shame resulting from an offence; their approval of significant others who are law abiding; and their ability to distinguish 'appropriate' from 'inappropriate' targets for crime (Sykes and Matza, 1957: 666). Matza has argued that young people are 'in a limbo between convention and crime' (1964: 28), and choose through rationalization or neutralization to 'drift' along a continuum from constraint to freedom, because of a tendency to procrastinate in respect of commitment and decision-making. Crime is thus episodic and temporary rather than constant. Matza's (1964) concept of drift is important in helping to understand children and young people's conscious and pragmatic search for the capital associated with social integration and status, even though this capital may come from offending in the short term.

Conclusions

As described above, whilst theories of young people's reasons for reducing or stopping offending are increasing in number, most notably in the USA (Laub and Sampson, 2003; Shover, 1996) and the UK (Farrall, 2000; Farrall and Bowling, 1999; Jamieson *et al.*, 1999; Maruna, 2001), no research has been identified which has systematically compared young people's reasons for starting with those given for stopping offending and aligned these with youth transitions. The voices of young offenders themselves are also rarely heard in studies relating to criminological theory generally, although they are increasingly heard in more specific evaluations of criminal justice interventions *per se*.

Nevertheless, most of the theories referenced in this chapter support the proposition that social integration, whether this be by individual, structural or socio-political means, is an important factor influencing the behaviour and attitudes of young people in transition today. Most theorists agree that young people tend to be keen to adjust within society, to achieve their aspirations and to be recognized by society as a whole for their efforts (see, for example, Barnado's, 1996; Wallace, 1987). However, cultural, subcultural and other criminological theories on their own, whilst allowing a description and analysis of why young people may choose deviant means to conventional ends, do not take full cognizance of young people's expectations, aspirations and opportunities in relation to significant others during the transition to adulthood.

As criminological theory currently stands, there seems to be a lack of congruence and continuity between those factors influencing onset and those influencing desistance. On the one hand, socio-cultural determinants (structural constraints) tend to be seen as most influential in young people's propensity to start offending, and, on the other hand, individual determinants (agency) tend to be seen as most influential in young people's desistance from offending. Whilst socio-political correlates (if not causes) are associated with onset, regrettably no such socio-political 'solutions' are offered in the desistance literature, placing the emphasis more on the individual to reduce or stop offending. This anomaly – that marginalization is associated with onset but is not necessarily addressed in desistance – requires further attention. In order to assess the extent of congruity and continuity between starting and stopping offending and to examine offending as a process of change for young people, it seems imperative first to explore the position of young people in society more generally, their transitional experiences from childhood through youth to adulthood, and their relative lack of power and status during that transitional phase. The following chapter, therefore, briefly explores the literature on youth transitions and the notion of power and powerlessness during that transition.

Chapter 3

Power and powerlessness in transition

I think I've learnt ... I was just a wee laddie then. I'm now a young man. More the man I want to be.

(Derek, 21)

Introduction

As was suggested in Chapter 2, there are few criminological theories that are successful in fully understanding offending as a *process* of change for the individual in the transition to adulthood. By 'process' I mean that offending and non-offending combine to make up a series of interrelated actions through time and space to achieve a desired outcome. Offending is not, generally speaking, a lifelong phenomenon, since the vast majority of people who start offending also stop offending after a relatively short period in youth. Offending could thus be seen during this period as a means, however misguided, of achieving economic, social or personal ends. The short-term end result, for many of the young people in this book at least, was interaction and integration with others of similar age in the transition to 'adulthood'. Non-offending – following successful desistance – was a further means to an end, namely wider social integration.

It is argued here that combining criminological theory with youth transitions enables linkages and consistencies to be identified between the process of starting and stopping offending and the process of the transition to adulthood. Whilst theories of youth transitions (e.g. Coles, 1995; Jones, 1996; Wyn and White, 1997) cannot explain offending behaviour *per se*, they can help us understand offending and desistance as a process and demonstrate more fully the extent to which offending may help to rectify, in the short term, the unequal distribution of power for young people in transition. Given the emphasis within the desistance literature on employment and relationships as a stimulus to stopping offending, a parallel investigation of transitions (where employment and relationships are two key components) would also seem pertinent. Likewise, the widening debate over the need to combine agency and structure in the criminological literature (Farrall and Bowling, 1999) has commonalities with more recent youth transitions research highlighted in this chapter. Before exploring youth transitions research more fully, the following section first examines broader anthropological literature relating to 'rites of passage' which have relevance to the concept of youth transitions.

The liminal status of youth

The terms 'youth' and 'youth transitions' are concepts which have attracted increasing sociological interest since the 1980s in understanding the extended and fragmented period that young people may go through before attaining full 'adult' status (Chisholm, 1993; Coles, 1995). The term 'youth' has become an additional stage between childhood and adulthood to exemplify this protracted transition (see, for example, Bynner *et al.*, 1997). However, prior to this increasing sociological interest in youth transitions, anthropologists had been examining the experiences of adolescents in small-scale societies and the 'rites of passage' that they progress through in preparation for adulthood. Whilst the term 'youth' was not seen as a middle phase between childhood and adulthood in such anthropological studies, Van Gennep (1960, cited in Turner, 1967) nevertheless identified three elements in the transition from childhood to adulthood in terms of 'rites of passage'. These are:

- *separation* – 'symbolic behaviour signifying the detachment of the individual or group either from an earlier fixed point in the social structure or a set of cultural conditions (a "state")';
- *margin* – 'during the intervening "liminal" period, the characteristics of the ritual subject (the "passenger") are ambiguous; [s/he] passes through a cultural realm that has few or none of the attributes of the past or coming state';
- *aggregation* – 'the passage is consummated. The ritual subject... is in a stable state once more and, by virtue of this, has rights

and obligations of a clearly defined and "structural" type' (Turner, 1967: 94–5).

Whilst Van Gennep focused on the more positive aspects of 'ritual' and 'ceremony' for young people in making the transition to adulthood, his middle 'liminal' phase has been adapted here to emphasize the more negative interpretations of youth which have been usurped by governments to restrict or forestall young people's movements as full citizens. The rites of passage of girls and young women in different cultures tended to be played down in this anthropological literature, although the liminal period was often described in terms of stereotypical feminine traits such as weakness and passivity. Turner (1969) describes individuals within the liminal phase as: 'persons or principles that (1) fall in the interstices of social structure, (2) are on its margins, or (3) occupy its lowest rungs' (ibid.: 125). Cloward and Ohlin (1961: 55) also see adolescence as a crucial marginalizing phase in the transition to adulthood: '... male adolescents are cut off from adult roles and relegated to a prolonged preparatory status in which they are no longer children but are not yet adults'. Whilst these authors were speaking some forty years ago along with their counterparts in anthropology, the status of young people in transition has changed little in the interim, and arguably has deteriorated.

Whilst the term 'youth' has more recently offered a sociological bridge between the widening poles of childhood and adulthood in the Western world, the phase of 'youth' is more than the 'liminal' phase described in the rites of passage literature. As James and Prout (1997) suggest, growing up nowadays involves several transitional processes rather than a one-off initiation process: youth transitions extend 'over considerable periods of time rather than being concentrated into ritual moments' (ibid.: 248). Nevertheless, it is in the late teens and early twenties that many people experience discrimination, socially, legally and economically, as a direct result of their age, and hence their status as 'liminal beings'.

The phases of transition

MacDonald and Marsh (2005) suggest that much criminal career research is overly deterministic and positivistic and that it would benefit from also considering the wider experiences of young people in transition. Whilst youth transitions research has not been used systematically in the field of criminology to date, these authors argue that such literature can provide a better understanding of youth offending as perceived and experienced by young people themselves. Not only are the phases of transition important markers to young people, but they should also be important markers to criminologists keen to understand the usually temporary and youthful nature of offending. Studying youth transitions in parallel with youth offending enables an exploration of the dynamics of age, power, interdependence and integration in the transition to full citizenship in adulthood.

Youth transitions research tends to adhere to a differentiation of the various phases of transition by chronological age, namely, 'childhood' (0–14), 'youth' (15–24) and 'adulthood' (25+) (see, for example, Jones, 1996). It is acknowledged that these transitional phases, like those of onset, maintenance and desistance used in this book, are zigzagging, overlapping and contentious, and as such, are merely heuristic devices, used as markers of change or development for children and young people. The factors which do, however, differentiate them one from the other are described briefly below.

Childhood

Childhood as a distinct and separate phase in the lifecycle was seen to emerge in the seventeenth century to distinguish children from their older counterparts (Aries, 1962). Aries's seminal work on childhood, although based on minimal empirical data and using modern (and masculine) conceptions of childhood (Archard, 1993; Wiltshire, 2003, pers. comm.), was nevertheless influential in its time in suggesting that children needed to be protected for moral as well as educational reasons. Aries (1962: 412) described children as being 'subjected to a special treatment, a sort of quarantine', and even though recent Children's Acts and the UN Convention on the Rights of the Child have attempted to diffuse the sense of 'quarantine', the term 'childhood' still differentiates children from adults in terms of risk, protection and rights and emphasizes the 'otherness' of children (Brown, 1998; Franklin, 2002). Children are increasingly given legal and protected status which separates them out from their older counterparts and which both enables and restricts their access to rights and responsibilities as citizens (Barry, 2001a). Children are almost totally dependent in a legal sense on adults, in particular on their families or carers, but once they reach school age, this dependence on families dissipates (albeit often temporarily) as the school milieu takes over, not only in terms of education and daytime supervision but also for leisure and social interaction. It is within the school environment that children increasingly relate to other children rather than family for leisure, identity and companionship. For many children from disadvantaged communities, 'childhood' does not offer the same type of protection that it offers young people from more affluent communities, against, for example, poverty, marginalization or taking on responsibilities as carers, thus questioning the traditional image of childhood as being a time of innocence and protection.

Youth

As mentioned above, the term 'youth' is a relatively new sociological concept, and indeed it was only in the eighteenth century that changing social conventions and tighter social legislation *'made* the adolescent' (Musgrove, 1964: 34, emphasis in original). The term 'youth' has now come to exemplify the extended transition from childhood to adulthood as a result of increasing restrictions on school leavers within the labour market as well as the commodification of this section of the population by consumer and other markets (Roberts, 2003). According to Coles (1995: 4), youth is 'an interstitial phase' between childhood and adulthood, during which young people are treated 'neither as children nor as adults' (ibid.: 6). Musgrove (1964) is more specific in suggesting that youth is an oppressed group, rejected by adults, and that young people's exclusion from 'adulthood' has been engineered for adverse rather than benign reasons.

Youth could be described as a time of distancing from, initially, the family environment and subsequently, the school environment, offering increased levels of autonomy and enabling experimentation with identities. The main milieu within which young people congregate is the friendship group, both within and outside the school environment, although many young people may still retain strong links with their families and the wider community during the youth phase.

The concept of 'youth' has been criticized for segregating and problematizing young people to the exclusion of the wider social and political environment of which they are a part. Jeffs and Smith (1998: 45) argue: 'that "youth" has limited use as a social category and that it characteristically involves viewing young people – mainly young men – as being in deficit, from a developmental perspective, and in need of training and control'. This is particularly apparent in relation to young offenders, who are being swept into a more punishment- and adult-oriented criminal justice system.

Adulthood

All individuals aged 25 and over are deemed to come under the rubric of 'adulthood', irrespective of their competence, since from that age all legal rights are in place (Jones, 1996). At the age of 25, individuals have full responsibilities as citizens, they are expected to support themselves through paid employment or other income, although they are also eligible for state benefits, and they are liable to pay taxes towards services for themselves and others. However, adulthood is not necessarily an 'end point' when specific rights and privileges are bestowed, but is a social construct dependent on social, legal, historical, cultural and personal contexts.

The key factors which young people equate with adulthood are parenthood, a home of one's own and stable employment, but these vary in importance for young people depending on social class and gender (Thomson and Holland, 2002). Adults are also more likely to interact with a wider social network, not least because of a wider range of contacts and commitments relating to employment, housing or child-rearing, and to have a greater power/influence over their own destiny because of increased equality and rights within the wider society.

Research on youth transitions

The advent in the UK of Thatcherism in the late 1970s marked a turning point not only for children and young people who became increasingly confined to the family and marginalized from the labour market, but also for sociologists of youth who had hitherto concentrated their attention on youth subcultures at the expense of structural constraints on youth transitions (MacDonald *et al.*, 2001). In an attempt to focus more on the socio-economic climate in which youth transitions took place, transitions research in the 1980s and early 1990s focused more on structural constraints than on individual choice. However, such research has more recently been criticized for being overly deterministic and throwing the proverbial baby out with the bath water in analysing the structure-agency debate. As Miles (2000: 10) argues:

> The tendency ... to adopt a structural perspective on transitions has been counter-productive, primarily because of its failure to prioritize the actual views, experiences, interests and perspectives of young people as they see them, in favour of bland discussions, most commonly of trends in employment and education patterns.

Traditionally, therefore, transitions research has portrayed a linear, psychosocial movement towards conventional goals. The main transitional pathways or 'careers' identified by such sociologists in the 1980s and early 1990s have been summarized by Coles (1995) as follows:

- the transition from full-time education and training to a full-time job in the labour market (the school-to-work transition);
- the transition from family of origin (mainly the biological family) to family of destination (the domestic transition);
- the transition from residence with parents (or surrogate parents) to living away from them (the housing transition).

Cohen and Ainley (2000: 81) suggest that the above categories of transition are no longer applicable to young people's position in society: 'education no longer relates necessarily to work, nor home-making to marriage or marriage to child-rearing'. Indeed, some say that transitions are no longer a youth phenomenon nor uni-directional, but apply to all people of all ages at different times. Roberts (2003: 6) suggests that: 'Most sociologists have abandoned trying to define youth in terms of chronological age. Nowadays we say that we study youth transitions which may occur at age 12, 16, 20, 30 or even when individuals are older than this'. He goes on to argue that 'Some people never establish themselves in jobs which will support an adult lifestyle. Some remain unmarried and childless, and continue to live in their parents' homes until the latter's death' (ibid.: 8).

Nevertheless, the period of youth – as in the age range 15–25 – is a time of life when there are major changes and decisions made which often impact irretrievably on young people's futures. Whilst for Turner's (1967; 1969) small-scale traditional societies referred to earlier, this period was a planned-for stage pending a 'new beginning', for many disadvantaged young people in Britain this phase in the lifecycle holds no status and there are few supportive structures to guide their transition to adulthood. This lack of support in the liminal phase leaves young people precariously poised between the two stools of protected children and autonomous adults (Barry, 2002).

The elements of transition described by, *amongst others*, Van Gennep and Coles are predominantly structurally defined and determined, whereas one further element less often cited in the youth transition literature is that of the transition from dependence to independence (Jones, 1996). This more individualized description of the transition phase allows young people's own narratives to come to the fore, and it is these narratives that have recently made academics question the linear approach to transitions which had hitherto been the norm. Stephen and Squires (2003), for example, argue that young people's transitions in late modernity are neither linear nor predictable but are fragmented, prolonged and cyclical. Equally, young people are increasingly seen as being proactive in defining, negotiating and making sense of their own transitions. Many recent accounts of young people's experience of youth transitions (*amongst others*, Holland *et al.*, 1999; Barry, 2001a and 2001b) suggest that their narratives and transitional experiences are guided as much by personal agency and responsibility as they are by structural factors.

According to Beck (1992), the certainties associated with industrial society have been eroded by a new age of modernity consisting of uncertain risks and opportunities, resulting in what he terms 'individualization'. This suggests that young people now have to resolve their own problems, overcome structural constraints and 'individualize' their own life projects (Cote, 2002). This fragmentation of past stability has resulted, in the last decade or so, in the transition research pendulum swinging away from structuralism and back towards a 'new freedom' of individualized lifestyles and reflexive construction of one's own biography (Holland *et al.*, 1999). Whilst the concept of individualization describes both structure and agency, the individual is nevertheless at the centre (albeit structurally defined), and factors such as class, gender and social networks are peripheral. Furlong and Cartmel (1997), however, warn against an over-emphasis on individualization at the expense of social and structural change, suggesting it would be an epistemological fallacy to focus on individual responsibility and self-determination without taking into account the powerful impact of existing social structures.

If, as Beck (1992) suggests, agency has superseded structure in youth transitions through the 'individualization' of young people, then it would seem reasonable to assume that the timing of such transitions would vary greatly between individuals, depending on their capacity to progress their life projects. Nevertheless, there tends to be a continuity in the overall timing of transitions, not least as illustrated by the age–crime curve, and this general continuity suggests that structural factors are more constraining than individual factors are enabling. Young people from disadvantaged backgrounds have had to resort increasingly to using agency (or more exactly 'entrepreneurial skills') in the transition to adulthood because of the presence of structural barriers. For example, MacDonald *et al.* (2001: 3.5) argue that transitions research needs to explore the 'alternative careers' adopted by many disadvantaged young people, such as criminal careers and parenting (Craine, 1997) or 'fiddly work' (MacDonald *et al.*, 2001: 3.5).

An ethos of individualization also tends to legitimate the marginalization of young people by the state (Wyn and White, 1997). Wyn and White argue that age is 'socially constructed, institutionalized and controlled in historically and culturally specific ways' (ibid.: 11). This social construction of age, and the impact of postmodern thinking regarding individualization, has lessened the impact of class inequalities and resulted in young people generally viewing failure in the transition to adulthood as a personal problem rather than a public issue (Bates and Riseborough, 1993). The developmental approach to both youth transitions, 'at risk' youth and offending behaviour by young people may have been usurped by the state to mask or legitimate structural inequalities. Such an approach places emphasis on the process of adolescent development which is seen as divorced from structural factors. Wyn and White conclude that the marginalization and criminalization of young people in particular is deliberate and sustained, a means of 'deflecting attention away from the structural reasons for poverty and unemployment' (ibid.: 135). Wyn and White (1997) also argue that disadvantaged young people should not be seen as any different from other age groups, having the same conventional goals as most people in society: '... in many cases the "resistance" exerted by "disadvantaged" young people is not necessarily *against* mainstream institutions but constitutes struggles for a place *within* them' (ibid.: 92, emphases in original).

Transitions research seems to have become preoccupied with the structure/agency dichotomy within an extended and increasingly adverse socio-economic environment. This preoccupation seems to be at the expense of the notion of power, citizenship and rights. The political and social power imbalances operating within our society, not least in the transition phase between childhood and adulthood, tend to be played down in favour of identifying localized structural constraints and individual choice at the expense of the macro-level issue of young people's rights in the transition to full citizenship. It is thus to the concept of power – or capital – that this discussion now turns.

The concept of capital

It has been suggested here that criminological theory alone cannot offer a comprehensive and all-encompassing approach to the mainly temporary nature of offending amongst a mainly transient section of a mainly youthful population. A broader, more dynamic approach is needed that depicts offending behaviour as a process of change and development amongst young people. This book deploys the concept of youth transitions to enable this more comprehensive and all-encompassing approach to be developed.

Criminological literature has hitherto emphasized blocked aspirations, subcultural association or the labelling and prejudice of the wider society, but has not specifically focused on the socio-legal constraints of disparities of power and participation of young people in transition. MacDonald and Marsh (2005) argue that subcultural theories are useful in understanding youth transitions, and by drawing on youth transitions in this book, subcultural affiliations amongst young people can be viewed as more political than individual, more transient than durable, and more interdependent than rebellious. Youth subcultural affiliations can offer a temporary reprieve in the transition to more sustainable and durable sources of power and reciprocity in adulthood. Equally, participation through consumerism often acts as a source of power where no other sources of power may exist in youth (Jones and Wallace, 1992). Offending is one means of acquiring such consumer power where no legitimate financial means are available.

Matza suggests that powerlessness is a key factor in producing drift and therefore delinquency: 'Being pushed around puts the delinquent in a mood of fatalism... In that condition he is rendered irresponsible' (Matza, 1964: 89). Such powerlessness, it could be argued, manifests itself in the transition phase of youth when young people fall between the two stools of relative protection as children and interdependence as adults. Whilst offending is not just a problem for young people but is also concentrated in communities and cultures more generally that are disempowered through increasing unemployment and poverty, powerlessness is perhaps most acutely felt by young people in transition, and offending is often an escape from such disempowerment (Ferrell and Sanders, 1995).

Power is not a concept reducible to one single definition; indeed its meaning differs according to the context in which it is used. For example, it can imply force, manipulation, authority and economic or political influence, and according to Haugaard (2002: 2): '[t]here will always be specific usages which are particularly suitable to certain theoretical projects'. In denoting the type of power available to individuals within their social world, Bourdieu utilizes the concept of capital, a term which goes back to the beginning of the twentieth century, notably in relation to 'social capital'.

The term 'social capital' has a chequered history and seems to have first arisen in the USA in 1916, when the schools reformer, Hanifan, coined the phrase to denote the 'good will, fellowship, sympathy and social intercourse among the individuals and families who make up a social unit' (Putnam, 2000: 19). Whilst Bourdieu appropriated the concept of capital in the 1970s in Europe, two North American sociologists, Coleman (1988) and Putnam (1993; 2000) have also given prominence to the concept of social capital. To Coleman, social capital combines rational action with social structure, includes obligations, trust, expectations, norms and information-sharing, and whilst productive, is not always benign: 'A given form of social capital that is valuable in facilitating certain actions may be useless or even harmful for others' (Coleman, 1988: 98). Coleman suggests that social capital allows individuals to 'establish relations purposefully and continue them when they continue to provide benefits' (ibid.: 105). He thus infers that if social capital is proving more damaging than beneficial, then that particular source of social capital will cease to be utilized. However, Coleman's interpretation of social capital is rational and utilitarian

– he stresses the 'indebtedness' aspect of such capital rather than the social aspect.

Following on from Coleman's communitarian interpretation of social capital, Putnam (2000) identified four strands of social capital as follows: 1) civic community networks; 2) a 'sense of belonging' to a civic community; 3) norms of reciprocity and trust; and 4) positive attitudes towards, and engagement in, voluntary, state and personal networks (Morrow, 1999). More recently, he has identified two sub-categories of social capital: bonding social capital (exclusive and inward-looking group identities) and bridging social capital (inclusive and outward-looking group identities): 'Bonding social capital constitutes a kind of sociological superglue, whereas bridging social capital provides a sociological WD-40' (Putnam, 2000: 23). Again, he acknowledges the adversarial as well as the consensual impact of both types of capital. Webster *et al.* (2004: 30) also comment on the adversarial nature of some sources of bonding social capital, which can 'exclude, marginalize, constrain and entrap' young people. MacDonald and Marsh (2005), who worked closely with Webster and colleagues on a recent study of young people's transitions in Northern England, talk of 'the paradox of networks' (ibid.: 203), where poorer areas are seen as lacking bridging social capital but are nevertheless a major source of support and legitimate opportunities for young people. They quote Kearns and Parkinson (2001: 2105) who argue that because people from more disadvantaged communities tend to draw on bonding rather than bridging social capital within such communities, they can only 'get by' rather than 'get on'. MacDonald and Marsh also point out the negative influences of social networks amongst dependent heroin users and their greater need for bridging social capital beyond the milieu of their drug-using peers.

Putnam, like Coleman (1988), argues that social capital is both the individual and collective face of reciprocal social relations. It can be both 'warm and cuddly' and 'malevolent, antisocial' (Portes and Landolt, 1996: 21–2), depending on whether such capital's support, cooperation, trust and institutional effectiveness are aimed at positive or negative outcomes. However, Putnam's concept of social capital is seen as inappropriate to the experiences of young people, not least because young people tend to be excluded from civic participation and develop their own individualized social networks (Morrow, 2001; Raffo and Reeves, 2000). Morrow (2001: 55) argues that Putnam's concept is 'a woolly, catch-all category' and ignores the historical and economic context, is gender-blind (in that women's employment goes against the romanticized ethos of community), is culturally specific to the USA only and tends to ignore individual agency and one's capacity to generate one's own social capital. Morrow (2001: 54) further argues that these individualized social networks are more important to young people than communities *per se*:

> For children and young people, 'community' is more often a 'virtual' community of friends based around school, town centre and street, friends' and relatives' houses, and sometimes homes in two different towns, rather than a tightly-bound easily-identifiable geographical location.

Bourdieu's theory of social practice

With the bad press associated with the broader concept of capital, it is perhaps surprising that the work of the French sociologist, Pierre Bourdieu, has attracted so much attention in sociological and educational circles, although little to date in criminological circles. Bourdieu is principally interested in the *relational* context of everyday actions and perceptions: the struggle for identification and recognition (Bourdieu, 1989; May, 1996), a major resource for which is capital. Bourdieu attempts to bridge the gap in social theory between agency and structure, without losing the 'major contribution of the structuralist legacy to social science' (May, 1996: 125). The disciplines contained within the social sciences have long argued that there is a dichotomy between what Callinicos (1999: 79) has described as 'the anti-humanist dissolution of the subject practised by structuralism and post-structuralism... [and] the reduction of social structures to emanations of individual subjectivity common to both Rational Choice Theory and the phenomenological tradition'. Bourdieu (1990) suggests that individual and collective constructions of the social world are not developed in a vacuum but are reproduced by, and themselves reproduce, social structures and are thus subjected to structural constraints. There is a constant interplay between structural constraints and individual choice, and the importance of time, space, agency and the individual's capacity to change are all implicated in the construction and reconstruction of the social world (Bourdieu, 1990).

Bourdieu's theory of social practice (1986) stresses personal networks and focuses as much on agency and sociability as on structure and institutionalization as well as on power relationships and the inevitability of the unequal distribution of capital amongst different groups and societies. Bourdieu argues that throughout their lives, individuals accrue capital – social, cultural, economic and symbolic – through their social practice (Bourdieu, 1984). These forms of capital, as utilized by Bourdieu, are described in more detail below.

Social capital is defined by Bourdieu (1997: 51) as:

> the aggregate of the actual or potential resources which are linked to possession of a durable network of more or less institutionalized relationships of mutual acquaintance and recognition – or in other words, to membership in a group – which provides each of its members with the backing of the collectively-owned capital, a 'credential' which entitles them to credit.

In other words, social capital is valued relations with significant others and is generated through relationships which in turn bring resources from networks and group membership. To Bourdieu, social capital includes not only social networks but also 'sociability' – 'a continuous series of exchanges in which recognition is endlessly affirmed' (1986: 250). As will be seen from the stories of the young people in this book, social capital gained within the peer group is a crucial source of support and recognition for young people in transition.

Economic capital is the financial means to not only the necessities but also the luxuries of everyday living, including inheritance, income and assets. Bourdieu stresses the dominance of economic capital in the market place because such capital can be transmitted, preserved and rationally managed (Bourdieu, 1990). Economic capital is not a major source of capital for young people generally, given their transient status between childhood and adulthood, their confinement to full-time education and their resulting segregation from the adult labour market, although it is acknowledged that young people from middle class backgrounds will be able to draw more readily on the economic and other capitals accruing from their families. For young people who have few responsibilities or commitments, economic capital may bring short-term status rather than longer-term financial security. However, for those offenders who commit crime as a means of earning a living, which Stewart *et al.* (1994: 19) refer to as 'professional' offenders, a successful criminal career may be consciously chosen as a viable alternative source of economic capital to employment.

Cultural capital is legitimate competence or status and comes from knowledge of one's cultural identity in the form of art and education in particular: 'language use, manners and orientations/ dispositions... and formal qualifications' according to Jenkins (1992: 116). It exists in three forms – in an embodied state of long-lasting dispositions of mind and body (e.g. styles and modes of presentation and identity); in an objectified state, as in cultural goods; and in an institutionalized state, through educational and other qualifications or status. To Bourdieu, cultural capital is not easily acquired or transmitted and is seen as an established form of capital that only truly gains legitimacy over time and via institutionalized or objectified means. It does not lend itself readily, therefore, to the relatively short (in terms of the lifecycle) transition period between childhood and adulthood.

Symbolic capital, to Bourdieu, is an overarching resource that brings prestige and honour gained from the collective, legitimate and recognized culmination of the other three forms of capital (Bourdieu, 1989): 'Capital has to be regarded as legitimate before it can be capitalized upon' (Skeggs, 1997: 8). Symbolic capital is 'the power granted to those who have obtained sufficient recognition to be in a position to impose recognition' (Bourdieu, 1989: 23), and is primarily accrued through: 'services, gifts, attention, care, affection' (Bourdieu, 1991: 128). It is, in effect, the 'recognition' received from a group:

> ... struggles for recognition are a fundamental dimension of social life and... what is at stake in them is the accumulation of a particular form of capital, honour in the sense of reputation and prestige, and ... there is, therefore, a specific logic behind the accumulation of symbolic capital, as capital founded on cognition [*connaissance*] and recognition [*reconnaissance*].
> (Bourdieu, 1990: 22, emphases in original)

However, Bourdieu argues that symbolic capital is basically unstable in comparison with economic capital: 'being based on reputation, opinion and representation ... [it] can be destroyed by suspicion and criticism, and is particularly difficult to transmit and to objectify' (Bourdieu, 1990: 93).

Field, habitus and practice

In an attempt to bridge the gap between structure and agency, Bourdieu utilizes three key underlying concepts in his theory of social practice, namely field (objectivity), habitus (subjectivity) and practice (interaction). Jenkins (1992: 85) defines a *field* as 'a network, or a configuration, of objective relations between positions objectively defined ... a structured system of social positions'. Fields are the site of struggles between holders of capital and are constituted by the distribution of different types of capital or power within them: they reflect the 'unequal distribution of capital' (Bourdieu, 1986: 46).

Habitus is both 'an internalization of reality' and, through practice, 'an externalization of self as constituted through past experience' (Haugaard, 2002: 225). Habitus is the unconscious shaping of actions and interactions and can change over time. The habitus bridges the gap between history and sociology in that it is 'history embodied in human beings' (May, 1996: 126), but external circumstances interplay with individual practice to create expectations and aspirations; individuals cannot of themselves influence how or when external circumstances change. This makes habitus seem like a self-fulfilling prophecy, and hence lays Bourdieu open to the criticism of being overly deterministic (Jenkins, 1992).

Finally, *practice* is the conscious result of the interplay between habitus and field. Whilst practice is often unquestioned – as interaction, behaviour or everyday life – Bourdieu attempts to construct a theoretical model of social practice (Jenkins, 1992). Social practice is not merely what people say and do, but why, when and where they say and do it. The interplay between the habitus (agency or subjectivity) and the field (structure or objectivity) results in a congruence between the individual and his/her social world that makes the latter seem self-evident and thus acceptable to the individual.

The methods by which individuals accrue capital within their practice are predominantly strategic. To Bourdieu, strategies are an important link between fields, habitus and practice, even though the habitus is mainly made up of 'tacit' knowledge. To Bourdieu, strategies are less rigid and circumscribed than rules, and include rational calculation (tempered by the constraints of limited resources) and the achievement of objectives in the medium to long term (Jenkins, 1992). However, strategizing is not only about rational choice but incorporates the needs/expectations of significant others. Bourdieu describes it as 'a feel for the game: a practical sense' which emanates from the habitus (Fowler, 2000: 77).

The durability and legitimacy of capital

The concepts of durability and legitimacy are crucial to an understanding of the effects of capital accumulation on the individual or group in society and will be discussed further in Chapter 7. Meantime, these two concepts are described briefly below in relation to the significance of capital accumulation for young people in transition.

Capital of whatever kind takes time and effort to accumulate and to transmit. Its potential for profit and reproduction is therefore, through time, dependent on the structure, dynamics and constraints of the social world (Bourdieu, 1986). *Durability* is an important element in Bourdieu's concept of capital. He describes social capital as being a 'durable network' (1997: 51) and recognition as being a 'durable feeling' (1998: 102). However, whilst social, cultural, economic and symbolic capital are readily identifiable forms of potential power for young people, it is argued here that for many young people *in transition*, they are not durable, not least because they are not recognized as legitimate by the wider society as a result of the paucity of opportunities available at this stage in their lives.

Capital thus takes on a less durable profile in relation to young people who are in transition. Young people, by dint of their status as 'transitional beings' (Turner, 1967: 98) and especially those from working class backgrounds, tend to have few, if any, fixed or permanent obligations towards, responsibilities for, or expectations of gaining capital beyond their immediate environment of friends and family. Durability of capital, along with collective legitimacy (see below) is one of the crucial elements that is missing within the childhood and youth phases, partly because of young people's liminal state both economically and socially, but also because they are not seen as full citizens with the longer-term obligations, independence and responsibilities associated with adulthood (Jones, 1995). Turner (1967: 100), in describing the 'liminal phase' – albeit in relation to primitive societies but arguably of relevance in modern society – has identified equality as being a strong factor in relationships between individuals in transition: 'The liminal group is a community or comity of comrades'. Turner argues that this equality is based on a negation, amongst young people in transition, of the factors which characterize status in society:

> transitional beings... *have* nothing. They have no status, property, insignia, secular clothing, rank, kinship, position, nothing to demarcate them structurally from their fellows.
> (Turner, 1967: 98–9, emphasis in original)

Bourdieu's definition of *legitimacy* is sociological rather than legal and refers to recognition and acceptance more than to authority and compliance. Sennett and Cobb (1972: 265) suggest that legitimacy is related to 'social rights': 'the source of social legitimacy in capitalist society comes primarily from what a person produces... and who he essentially *is*' (ibid.: 267–8, emphasis in original). It is one's identity rather than what one produces that is the key to Bourdieu's understanding of legitimacy. Bourdieu defines 'legitimacy' as '[a]n institution, action or usage which is dominant, but not recognized as such, that is to say, which is tacitly accepted' (Bourdieu, 1984: 110). In other words, capital of whatever form is legitimate or 'symbolic' only in an implied sense. The concept of legitimacy is important in the gaining and imposition of symbolic capital. Symbolic capital accrues when one's actions or power are acknowledged, legitimated and finally recognized but since, to Bourdieu, the nation state 'is the site par excellence of the concentration and exercise of symbolic power' (Bourdieu, 1998: 47), it is less effective in a 'restricted market' (Fowler, 2000: 41) where official legitimation is unlikely outside of the 'mainstream'.

Capital accumulation in transition

Whilst Bourdieu infers that the accumulation of symbolic capital requires both durability and *official* legitimacy within the wider society, I argue that for young people in transition, in the possible absence of other forms of capital, symbolic capital is also a viable and vital source of identity, status, recognition, reputation and power within the friendship group and although not necessarily durable, can accrue once legitimated by other young people in the short term rather than by the wider society in the longer term. Such 'informal' legitimation could offer children and young people from disadvantaged backgrounds improved access to continuity and recognition in an otherwise decompartmentalized and potentially unstable set of transitional experiences and networks.

The discussion in this book is based on an appropriation of various of Bourdieu's concepts in order to demonstrate the possible relationship between the phases of offending and those of transition. It could be argued, for example, that Bourdieu's concept of field could apply equally to the constructs of childhood, youth and adulthood, in that these phases of transition are 'a structured system of social positions' (Jenkins, 1992: 85) embedded within age- and status-determined power relations within society. Bourdieu (1986: 46) suggests that the field reflects an 'unequal distribution of capital' and indeed, in the analysis used in this book, the forms, sources and levels of capital accumulation vary between each phase of transition, depending on the value placed on such capital by both the holders of it and those significant others who contribute towards, or restrict, its accumulation. Bourdieu also suggests that the habitus may become torn between two or more fields, resulting in the possibility of heterodoxy or orthodoxy (May, 1996) – respectively, an undermining or an acceptance of the status quo. Offending behaviour in childhood and youth could be argued to be a manifestation of heterodoxy, whilst desistance in adulthood could be argued to be a manifestation of orthodoxy, based on a redistribution of capital. The internalization of new norms and values by young people, their progression through the fields of transition and the accumulation of different and extended forms of capital in adulthood can enable the modification of the habitus and the eventual orthodoxy of practice.

Table 3.1 demonstrates the various ways in which young people can accumulate capital *through conventional means*, whilst still acknowledging that capital can also be accumulated through offending. These conventional sources of capital for young people in transition are deduced both from Bourdieu's definitions of each type of capital and from the literature on youth transitions (for example, Coles, 1995; Jones, 1995) and youth culture (Brake, 1985; Miles, 2000; Willis, 1990). Such sources of capital are pertinent, but not necessarily available, to *all* young people, depending on the ease with which they can make the transition to adulthood, both from an agency and a structural perspective.

The analysis in the following chapters is based on the experiences, views and aspirations of the young people in this study. Case study

Table 3.1 Potential sources of conventional capital accumulation for young people

Capital	Onset/childhood	Maintenance/youth	Desistance/adulthood
Social	Family, friends	Friends, relationships	Family, wider social networks
Economic	Family income	Personal income	Employment
Cultural	Schooling	Consumption, acquisition of skills and qualifications	Further education
Symbolic	Family, friends, dependence	Friends, reputation, independence	Family, interdependence

material is drawn upon to illustrate the linkages between offending and transition and the relevance of capital. The case studies were chosen because they represent a cross-section of the overall sample in terms of age ranges and lengths of offending history. They also represent two ends of the spectrum in terms of desistance and persistence, in order to compare the varying levels of capital accumulation in the transition to adulthood and to explore these young people's levels of capital expenditure. Each respondent's classification of himself/herself as a 'persister' or 'desister' at the time of interview is acknowledged at the start of each case study.

Their reasons and explanations for offending at onset (Chapter 4), in the maintenance phase (Chapter 5) and in the desistance phase (Chapter 6), were subsumed under four different categories, which illustrate these young people's interpretation of their offending behaviour. These categories are: relational, monetary, practical and personal. Relational reasons include interactions with others whether such interactions are positive or negative. Monetary reasons include the need for money for general or specific purposes, e.g. survival, consumables or drugs. Practical reasons pertain to structural or external factors, such as the 'hassle factors' resulting from offending and its detection, health reasons and the employment and education implications of procuring a criminal record. Personal reasons relate to the individual's own needs and feelings. Whilst these categories emerged naturally from the primary analysis, it was found subsequently that these categories closely matched the concepts of capital espoused by Bourdieu described above, namely social, economic, cultural and symbolic capital. Whilst the analysis in the following chapters remains primarily true to the voices of the young people participating in the research, Bourdieu's interpretation is interspersed with the young people's perceptions in order to illustrate the potential of the concept of capital in understanding offending in transition.

Chapter 4

Starting offending

> No one cared. That's what I thought. There wasn't very much for me at that time. It was just me and me alone. And then I started getting in with the wrong crowd, older lassies ... I was acting big ... it was an ego boost.
>
> (Yvonne, 25)

Introduction

The criminological literature on offending implies that *starting* and *maintaining* offending are, in effect, two sides of the same coin. This study purposefully challenged this assumption by asking the same young people to attempt to differentiate between their experiences and perceptions of starting, continuing and stopping offending, albeit retrospectively, in order to unpick the process of change that occurs during those offending histories. The differences described in the following three chapters hopefully suggest that drawing such a distinction – between, most importantly, starting and maintaining offending – highlights the crucial differences in that process of change.

Their reasons and explanations for offending, both at onset and in the desistance phase (Chapter 6), were subsumed under four different categories cited in the previous chapter to illustrate the young people's interpretation of their offending behaviour. To reiterate, these categories were: relational, monetary, practical and personal. Relational reasons include interactions with others whether such interactions are positive or negative. Monetary reasons include the need for money for general or specific purposes, e.g. survival, consumables or drugs. Practical reasons pertain to structural or external factors, such as the 'hassle factors' resulting from offending and its detection, health reasons and the employment and education implications of procuring a criminal record. Personal reasons relate to the individual's own needs and feelings.

The impetus to starting offending

The criminological literature suggests that offending tends to start in early adolescence, with a peak age of onset of offending for both sexes at 14 or 15 (Farrington, 1995; Rutter *et al.*, 1998). Thirty-two of the young people in the study sample (18 men and 14 women) suggested at interview that they had started offending under the age of 15, with nearly two thirds starting between the ages of 12 and 15. Most of the young people suggested that starting offending was something that 'just happened' with only seven young men and five young women considering that they had made an active decision to do so, mainly at a later age and for financial reasons (e.g. for drugs or money generally).

> I said to myself, I'm going to need to have to go out and shoplift to support my habit.
>
> (Vicky, 27, started offending aged 22)

> It was pretty much my decision, yeah ... Well it was because I'd left my job, I was put in a situation that I was back in [town], I wasn't going to get a job outwith [town]. My brother, he always had money and he was always, had some form of drugs on him and he was always getting drunk and the only way that he could get money was like from crime, so I came to the conclusion that I'm not going to get the job I want ... so I need money and I had a lot of time on my hands so I needed to do something with myself and the only way I could get money was by breaking the law.
>
> (Martin, 24, started offending aged 18)

Personal or relational need, on the other hand, was the predominant reason for drifting into offending, with the influence of friends and immaturity being cited as precursors to starting offending:

It was just, there was a few of us about ... I think it was just I
was young, know what I mean ... friends have got something to
do with it ... if you're on your own, you wouldn't.

(Tom, 19, started offending aged 11)

... we used to go into town every weekend and, I mean a good
few of my friends were doing it before, I was always 'no, no, no,
no' ... I was getting called chicken and this and that ... and then
eventually I just thought, I'm not taking this any more, and just
went ahead and done it.

(Bernadette, 23, started offending aged 14)

Brown (1998) implies that women have greater difficulty than
men in committing crime because they are under greater surveillance
and control within the family and are more influenced to adopt
conventional, submissive or caring roles. As will be seen later in
this chapter, Sutherland and Cressey's (1970) theory of differential
association seemed to apply more readily to the women in the onset
phase, when they suggested that they 'learnt' to offend through the
tutelage of their (often older) peers or boyfriends.

Type of initial offence

Several authors have noted that the age of onset of offending differs
with different offence types (LeBlanc and Frechette, 1989; Jamieson
et al., 1999). Farrington (1997) has suggested that the age of onset
for shoplifting and vandalism, for example, tends to be younger,
on average at age 11, whereas the age of onset for burglary and
car theft is more likely to be 14–15, and for sex offences and drug
offences later still at age 16–17. However, it is unclear from this
literature whether one actively chooses an offence type or is driven
more by circumstances, irrespective of age.

Rutter *et al.* (1998) suggest that theft (including shoplifting) is
the most common offence committed by adolescents and Cunneen
and White (2002) also suggest that shoplifting is one of the largest
categories of offences for which children and young people are
apprehended. Certainly in this study, shoplifting was the most
prevalent *initial* offence committed by both young men (10/20) and
young women (15/20). Theft other than shoplifting (5/20 men and
1/20 women) and assault (3/20 men and 3/20 women) were equal
second in popularity as an initial offence. Given that many of the

respondents suggested that they started offending in the company of friends as a means of gaining attention or consolidating those friendships, many also suggested that shoplifting was a convenient offence to commit in this respect. Not only were shops readily accessible (often being passed on the way to or from school), but also they offered immediate gratification, in terms of visibility by friends and access to free consumables:

> It was just maybe a couple of cream eggs or a couple of bars of chocolate and going out to your mates and going 'look what I've got, whey hey!'. 'Get back in and get more'. But I wasn't realizing at the time, it was me that was going to get into all the bother for it and they're sitting outside eating it and I'm going back and getting more for them ... Crazy!
>
> (Carol, 29)

Whilst shoplifting has been traditionally seen as the preserve of female offenders, men are proportionately twice as likely as women to shoplift (Buckle and Farrington, 1984). This could be in relation to convictions rather than self-report data, since men are more likely to be the focus of attention by security staff in shops, given the accepted role of women as the main buyers of consumables. Theft other than shoplifting tended to be the first offence for those who started at a younger age (three of the six men who started offending under the age of 12 suggested that their first offence was housebreaking, and rarely did they go on to shoplifting later in their offending histories).

It has been suggested that the use of drugs rarely precedes the onset of offending, although the use of alcohol and tobacco does (Pudney, 2002), with the average age of onset for crime generally being 14.5 years compared to 16.2 years for illicit drug use and 13.8 years for alcohol. Pudney also suggests that there is a progression in both drug use and offending from minor to more serious activity. The offence of assault was often preceded by excessive alcohol intake amongst the sample, and those whose initial offences included assaults rarely went on to commit thefts in the future, tending to accrue instead additional convictions for breach of the peace, police assault and vandalism charges. Whilst the majority started off with minor offences of shoplifting or theft, their level and seriousness of offending (and drug use) increased markedly over the course of their offending histories, and these changes will be explored further in Chapter 5.

Factors influencing the onset of offending

During the interview, respondents offered various reasons as to why they had started offending and what had influenced them at that time. Their responses were, to some extent, interchangeable between the rationale for starting to offend and those events or people that might have had some influence or power over their propensity to start offending. The main factors influencing these young people were relational, mainly friends or siblings, personal, such as the excitement of offending, and monetary, the desire for money either for consumables or drugs.

Relational factors

Relational factors featured most prominently, although personal and monetary factors were almost as important explanations. Whilst a few (mainly young men) were influenced by their siblings who were offending – 'My big brother ... the two of us, we were like a team, you know ... we can take on armies' (Martin, 24) – the majority felt the need to 'follow the crowd', either to be seen to be sociable or to gain a sense of 'belonging' through identity with friends. In childhood, most of the young people's sources of social capital came from family and friends, although the levels of stability within their family and friendship groups varied dramatically. Many of these young people suggested that their family upbringings had *not* been a source of support or encouragement for them, resulting in them often turning to friends for company and social identity. Peer groups have a long-established link with one's propensity to offend (Reiss, 1988). Many authors acknowledge this link but suggest there is a lack of evidence of a causal, as opposed to correlational, relationship between peers and offending (Warr and Stafford, 1991; Rutter *et al.*, 1998). Rutter *et al.* (1998) state that negative peer influences in adolescence are most likely when individuals spend a lot of time in close proximity to other young people and where the group overtly approves of and encourages deviant activity.

It has been argued (Scottish Office, 1998; Stewart *et al.*, 1994) that young men are more likely to offend for sociable reasons than are young women, and that young women are restrained by the wider condemnation that offending might involve. However, Emler *et al.* (1987) suggest that female offenders are more likely than their male counterparts to offend in a group setting. The findings from my study support Emler *et al.* in respect of the social side of offending, as highlighted by the numbers of young women citing relational factors and sociability as reasons for starting offending. Although numbers are small, the women were twice as likely as the men to cite attention from friends and family as being an impetus to their starting offending. Chodorow (1974, cited in Gilligan, 1982) has suggested that women gain social and self identity more through interaction with others than do men. A woman, according to Gilligan, comes 'to know herself as she is known, through her relationship with others' (ibid.: 12).

Sutherland and Cressey's differential association theory (1970) suggests that people learn to offend in a group setting that approves of, and condones, such behaviour. Although these authors do not make gender-specific claims regarding differential association, it may be the case that young women are more likely to want to learn to conform to the group because of their greater need than young men for social and self identity. Several of the women suggested an element of 'learning' to offend when they first started:

> My two older brothers [were offending]. I think I just seen what they done and thought 'I'll do that'.
>
> (Janet, 21)

> All my friends were going into town to shoplift and dressing smart with the clothes that they'd stole and at first I was always saying 'how could they do that? I wish I could do that'. And then ... I was in town with my friend and she was a bit older than I was and she stole herself a big shiny necklace. She said 'just do it ... it's easy', and I did, and it was easy.
>
> (Helen, 20)

> I started getting in with the wrong crowd and it was older people, so it was like they were telling me to go do things because I was the youngest.
>
> (Carol, 29)

However, several of the young men in the sample suggested that they felt under pressure to conform to peer group influences, mainly to be included in that circle of friends. Pete, for example, described the need for the capital accruing from the new social network of his peers, having been uprooted from the familiar milieu of his earlier childhood.

Pete, 19, desister

Pete suggested that he started offending when he was 10, having moved from a city to a rural community and into a new school, hence a change in his sources of social, cultural and symbolic capital. Because he knew nobody at the school, was depressed following a traumatic earlier childhood, was concerned by his mother's alcoholism and was therefore unhappy at home, he concluded at the age of 10 that offending was a possible means of being placed in care away from his mother. Offending was also a means of gaining social and symbolic capital: *'I was looking for, I suppose in a way, folk to look at me in a different light. For folk to think of me differently – to fit in, in a way … and to be noticed by my mother and stuff, you know, with her alcohol abuse, I was always like alone and it was very difficult to like, I don't know, to get on with anyone, you know … I was picked on at school. I tried to keep myself to myself and other folk don't like that and I was an outsider so they went out of their way to do, you know, and that was what the main problem was really … I had to make friends because I was alone in a strange countryside village with no one that I knew about me and it was like, how – what can I do? Where am I gonna turn, you know? And to me, [offending] was my only escape.'* Pete tried to adapt his habitus in his new environment through gaining the attention of his peers and to *'fit in'* as he described it – a source of both social and symbolic capital in an otherwise isolating existence. However, he found that infiltrating this potential social network through offending proved counterproductive: *' … it never [got me friends], it put me in a worse position … Folk my own age and that rejecting me, you know. They didn't want anything to do with me and that was the hardest part.'*

Although many respondents suggested that their unhappy childhood experiences had influenced their likelihood of starting offending, either because of a lack of care or attention within the family, latent anger or poverty, the majority also equated starting offending with the desire to be with and impress friends. Lacking the social and symbolic capital that comes through respect, responsibility and attention within the family, many of these young people turned to a new circle of potential friends within the school environment. Like Pete, they chose a strategy which they thought fitted with the norm of that environment, namely consumption, experimentation, rebellion, mimicry and assimilation. For the women, sexual relationships formed in their early teenage years were also a source of social and symbolic capital, often giving them the love and attention from boyfriends that was otherwise missing in their childhoods.

Anna, 21, persister

Anna said she started rebelling when she was 14, mainly because her parents were very strict and she had a very poor relationship with her mother: *'[MB: What would have helped you ... Around the age of 14?] If my mum and dad had been less possessive and let me do my own thing ... If I'd more love. I mean, if my mum and dad showed me love instead of just being strict ... If my mum had been a better mother to me.'* This lack of social capital through her family, coupled with a move of family home and bullying at school, resulted in Anna resorting to offending in order to gain and keep friends, even though she described them as *'a really wrong crowd'*. Her boyfriend at the time was into shoplifting to fund a drug habit, and she drifted into a similar lifestyle aged 15. Anna said that the advantages of starting offending were that she got money for drugs, it gave her friends and it was fun. Thus, she gained economic, social and symbolic capital that was hitherto missing from her life in childhood.

Not only did being 'one of the crowd' bring social networks and sociability, but also the status these young people attained from offending with peers suggested that such social capital was valued and legitimated. The women in particular gained social capital from offending with friends as well as gaining economic, cultural and symbolic capital from the status symbols of youth, for example through shoplifting designer clothes and other items. Skeggs (1997) has argued that a young woman's feminine embodied cultural capital (how she looks to others and feels about herself) is her only 'tradeable' commodity in youth, whereas when she gets older, she may have access to the capital accruing from relationships or motherhood.

Laura, 27, desister

Laura started offending on entering secondary school, partly because it gave her money and friends but also because her parents had separated at that point and she moved out of the family home to live with her then-boyfriend who shared a flat with drug addicts. She was working part-time in a shop at the age of 13 from where she stole large quantities of cigarettes which her boyfriend then sold on: *'I made thousands of pounds, you know, stealing from the shop.'* She put much of her vulnerability at that age down to her relationship with her mother, which had not been a source of capital for her as a child: *'If my mum hadn't separated, if my mum had any time for me, you know … I didn't get the help … There was a lot of hatred between me and my mum… I wasn't getting on with my mum. Not feeling loved really.'* The social and symbolic capital of having a boyfriend and the economic capital accruing from her success at offending both gave her the attention which was lacking in her life at that time.

For many, the initial impetus to offending was to form friendships and gain attention. As Yvonne said in the opening quotation to this chapter, offending with peers was 'an ego boost' when no one else in her life cared for or about her. Such phrases highlight the importance in childhood of social capital, however unconventionally acquired that capital might be. Nevertheless, the young women tended to be more influenced by relationships than friends *per se*, even if these relationships involved abuse or offending. For five of the young women, having a boyfriend who was offending was a crucial stimulus to beginning offending, not least when those boyfriends were encouraging them to take drugs – or, as one woman described it, 'training' them to offend. Whereas many of the men would not have been involved in relationships at the time they started offending (they tended to start offending earlier than the women), the women were more likely to be in a relationship *before* they became involved in offending. Whereas for the young men, being involved in a relationship might be an impetus to *stopping* offending, for the young women relationships were often the impetus to *starting* offending:

> [My first boyfriend] was a drug dealer and I admired him ... I fancied him and I thought he was cool because everybody respected him and all the people my age respected me because I was mucking about with this person ... I wanted the speed. I needed it.
>
> (Nina, 23)

In relation to drug-abusing women and crime, the literature suggests that offending for drugs is often partner-induced (Covington, 1985), even if that involvement in relationships was not originally for the purpose of obtaining drugs but for the relationship itself (Taylor, 1993). Nevertheless, as the need for drugs increased, obtaining such drugs became a mutual interest within the relationship and one that kept the relationship going even when the focus of the relationship perhaps changed, in the women's view, from being loving and caring to being utilitarian and abusive (Taylor, 1993). The impact of drugs on offending for these young people is explored further in Chapter 5.

Personal factors

Starting offending because it was fun, exciting and relieved boredom were factors almost wholly the preserve of the young men. Ferrell and Sanders (1995: 311) suggest that the 'adrenalin rush' from crime is often an end result in itself, and Katz (1988: 54) describes shoplifting as a 'magical' experience over and above any material gain arising from such theft. However, Ferrell (1993: 171) suggests that such seduction is also bound up with the 'the illicit acquisition of late capitalist consumer goods'. Whilst Knight and West (1975) found only a quarter of their sample of 18–19-year-olds cited fun or the relief of boredom as reasons for offending, Downes (1966) found these personal factors to be prevalent amongst the majority of young people in his experience. Any discrepancy in such findings may arise because of the point at which respondents are asked whether offending is 'fun', in terms of whether they are referring to the onset or maintenance phase and their age at interview. This highlights the importance of differentiating between these two phases of offending.

Eight of the men in this sample suggested they *started* offending because of the buzz or through boredom (and shoplifting tended to be their initial offence of choice), whilst none of the women suggested that excitement was a primary reason or influence. However, as mentioned above, the women tended to start offending at an older age than the men and it could also be that excitement and autonomy, according to Gilligan (1982), are more the preserve of men whilst relational factors are more the preserve of women. Nevertheless, not all the women started offending for relational reasons, with many suggesting that the personal trauma of abuse in the past or present was a trigger to their starting offending. Anger or depression resulting from abuse or bereavement was cited by eight women but only one man as an influence on their propensity to start offending:

> When I was younger I got interfered with. That's got a lot to do with it, with anger and that ... I was only four.
>
> (Alison, 20)

The young man who cited abuse as a child had a particular reason for choosing mainly sexual offending:

> I wanted to – I wanted to sort of like hurt people the way that I was hurt.
>
> (Owen, 18)

Certainly, many of these respondents talked about bad childhood memories of bereavement, reconstituted family structures, exclusion from school, being in care and physical and sexual abuse:

> Just the way I was passed about in children's homes.
>
> (Len, 26)

> ... just being moved from pillar to post ... mental and physical abuse ... From zero to sixteen, I'd just been thrown from pillar to post ... it made us tough, didn't it?
>
> (Nick, 28)

It was a horrible childhood ... my mum and dad split up when I was 14 – happiest day of my life when my mum and dad split up because she was just a punch bag to him. At the weekends she was his punch bag ... I think I was already off the rails by that time.

(Theresa, 33)

The gender difference in these personal factors, notably in relation to anger and loss, equates with one of Stewart *et al.*'s (1994) six category typology of reasons for offending, namely 'Self-expression' resulting from frustration, stress or anti-authority attitudes. Stewart *et al.* disagree with the suggestion made by Utting *et al.* (1993) that bereavement, for example, is not readily associated with offending, and argue that the loss of a family member – by whatever means (e.g. death or separation) – can be an extremely stressful 'critical moment' (MacDonald *et al.*, 2001) which can influence offending behaviour. Stewart *et al.* (1994) also note the more likely propensity of women to offend as a result of such loss, and revised strain theory (Katz, 2000) also suggests that women will be more likely to offend because of the anger resulting from childhood abuse or neglect. Yvonne's story epitomized that kind of stress.

Yvonne, 25, desister

Yvonne's mother left her father when Yvonne was 9, and Yvonne did not see her father again. Her mother and the seven children moved to Scotland, causing a break in Yvonne's sources of social capital in particular from wider family and friends. For the first few years things went well for Yvonne, but then her mother started drinking heavily when Yvonne entered her teens, thus restricting further her access to social capital: ' ... *my mum being an alcoholic and then she battered me. She couldn't be bothered. Going with all different men. She just didn't care. She was just going out drinking all the time.*' Yvonne turned to her peers for attention through offending at the age of 13. She also spent some time in care where she received the social, cultural and symbolic capital that was lacking in her earlier childhood: '*I got spoiled when I was in care. I was getting clothes bought for me, I was getting taken to*

> *places, but at my mum's, she wasn't caring. She wasn't buying us good clothes, nothing. She never took us anywhere. She never gave us any money or anything.'*

Just as getting older will be seen in Chapter 6 to have been a factor influencing desistance for some of this sample, getting older was also a factor influencing onset: no longer being seen as – or feeling like – a child gave one the opportunity to develop autonomy and increased self-identity within a wider social context:

> I wasn't going out and doing anything nasty but I was more nasty to my dad, like saying I'm not staying in and I'm not doing this and I'm not doing that and I was basically doing my own thing as I was getting older.
>
> (Carol, 29)

Monetary factors

The need for money (either for survival, consumables, drugs or alcohol) was often cited as a reason for starting to offend, but whereas the young men tended to want money for consumables, many of the young women started to offend because of their need to buy drugs, either for themselves or because of encouragement by their drug-using partners:

> It was just clothes and that ... able to get myself new clothes basically ... my mum [did] when she could, not when I wanted. [*MB: Was clothes the only thing that you really wanted the money for?*] Clothes, bikes, football kits and stuff.
>
> (Vic, 23)

> You need to buy in bulk when you're dealing because you need to make the profit, so I didn't have the money to do that, so I started shoplifting and any money I got I was just buying a bag, two bags [of heroin], whatever I could get. As my face got known for shoplifting, I stopped that and went into housebreaking.
>
> (Vicky, 27)

McIvor *et al.* (2004) note that whereas offending preceded drug use for the men in their sample of young people, drug use was the impetus to the women in that study starting offending, hence suggesting a strong link between offending and a lack of money for women. Bates and Riseborough (1993: 2) suggest that many young people live under 'the canopy of structured inequality' and Craine (1997: 136) also argues in his study of disadvantaged young people that: 'Although choices were made and individual biographies and careers constructed, these were frequently desperate survival adaptations ... not as they pleased, nor under circumstances of their own choosing'.

Whilst some of the respondents talked of offending to survive (for food, drugs or shelter), the majority wanted money as a means of self and social identity: to have the goods and status symbols that their peers had, as illustrated by Derek's story.

Derek, 21, persister

Derek suggested he came from a stable family background and that his relationship with his parents, brother and two sisters had always been good. He was one of the few young people in this study who spoke positively about their family background. At the age of 12 when he entered secondary school, he said he started offending (initially shoplifting and housebreaking) to keep in with and impress his friends. At that age he was of below average height, was bullied at school and felt the need to prove himself through the cultural and symbolic capital of being 'macho' and 'hard', traits which were an expected part of the youth culture of the area in which he lived: *'You just wanted to make a name for yourself ... I don't know. It's just about bottle. "I can do it, can you do it?" That's what it was like ... Well you wanted to offend with them. If you didn't, you'd feel left out ... you were in a group and that, and we just all done it. It was just, it's hard to explain. It's just spur of the moment when you're young and a boy, you don't think about it, you just do it.'* The social capital of his family was not enough to protect Derek from the wider environment of the area in which he lived and he was also conscious of the fact that he was not well-off compared with some of his friends. Keeping *in* with them also required keeping *up* with them: '*Well my mum and that never had much money. I was hanging about with a few pals that had money. They always had like a couple of pound and that was a lot in they days. But I mean, your mum and that's got a big family, ken, it's like that ... If my friends can buy it, I can get it for nothing, just like that ... I just wanted to be in there too. I didn't want to be the odd one out ... just reputation ... and to show that you can get it for nothing.*' The visibility of his offending with his peers, however, seemed to be more important to him than any utilitarian gain (economic capital) – the *showing* he could get it for nothing, rather than the actuality of getting it for nothing.

The cultural, social and symbolic power gained from offending was thus, to a certain extent, dependent on these young people's access to economic capital. Young women in particular may feel that their femininity or bodily image is their only asset, thus making the desire for designer clothes and accessories all the more important (Skeggs, 1997). One's 'style' epitomizes one's personal and group identity and is an essential element of collective behaviour, such as early offending with peers (Ferrell, 1995). But offending can not only provide the means of improving one's image, but also one's image can reflect opposition to the dominant culture. Style can thus be labelled as *potentially* criminal. As Ferrell (1995: 182) notes: 'In the lived experience of identity and inequality, personal and group style exists as a badge of resistance and honor' but it nevertheless can result in a spiral of criminalization, discrimination and amplification of such resistant behaviour.

Vic's story below epitomized the desire of these young people for economic capital and hence status. Vic was conscious of the poverty both of the area in which he lived and within his own family, and the fact that he could resort to offending for consumables was, to him, a direct consequence of that poverty.

Vic, 23, persister

Vic suffered physical abuse from the age of 3 from his stepfather, and was relieved when his mother left his stepfather when Vic was 10. He started stealing at the age of 8, the age when he suggested he started to 'register' what money really meant. However, he said he was the 'black sheep' in the family and was more influenced by the friends he was with at that time: ' ... *everyone else was doing it ... it was just the crowd I was hanging about with'*. He said he was more a follower than a leader and worried that if he did not join in their activities he would be left out or rejected by his friends. He suggested that offending was, therefore, a way to keep friends, a crucial source of social and symbolic capital to him at that time. He also realized that offending could be quite profitable, hence giving him additional economic capital. Although his mother bought him clothes, shoplifting enabled him to get what he wanted when he wanted, rather than when she could afford to buy them, and shoplifting clothes and football kit gave him both symbolic and cultural capital. He said the buzz and fun were also key ingredients in offending at that age: *'Just the buzz of getting away with it. And sort of showing off is a big part of it ... saying "I've more than you"'.* He suggested that many of his friends at that time were in residential care and he calculated that if he got caught, he may have been put into residential care, a further source of economic capital: *'They were getting 350 quid a month or something to get clothes. I thought I would get extra clothes ... They were getting taken to the pictures, skiing, things like that ... I thought, I want to go to that.'*

Many of the young people came from reconstituted or single-parent families and several had experienced periods of being looked after in residential settings. Whilst not implying that such an upbringing precludes one from accumulating capital within a family environment, it nevertheless often results in transient lifestyles or a lack of continuity of care and protection as children, which can have a major impact on one's ability to accumulate capital (Morrow, 2001). Emond (2000: 2), for example, suggests that being looked after has the double stigmatization of restricting contact with parents and of labelling the child as either 'troubled' or 'troublesome'. Whilst the majority of the respondents spoke of limited access to economic capital in childhood, one source of such capital was on entering the care system, as Vic acknowledged. Being 'looked after' gave one greater access to pocket money and new clothes as well as a social network with which one could readily identify.

Practical factors

Although funding the purchase of alcohol and drugs was cited as a factor that necessitated offending, several respondents also suggested that the effects of one or other substance also made offending more likely:

> Like, if I was drunk and stoned, I'd go and drive a car, fight the police and commit a breach of the peace, and maybe fight with somebody else.
>
> (Eric, 21)

> See when I was with amphetamines, it was like when I was on a come down, next day my mind would be totally different from that so I'd like go into a shop and I was feeling like I thought I was maybe invisible, that I could do it [shoplift].
>
> (Paula, 27)

Whilst some may have needed the 'Dutch courage' of alcohol or drugs in order to offend, many suggested that success was an influencing factor. Offending was something they could do relatively easily without getting caught, and 'getting away with it' was part of the attraction:

> ... once you start stealing and you get away with it, you think you're not going to get caught so you just go on stealing and stealing and every time you go into a shop you steal a little bit more.
>
> (Alec, 28)

Whilst only a minority specifically mentioned the ease with which they could offend as children, many more implied that their offending generally went undetected, suggesting at least some 'expertise' on their part or 'incompetence' on the part of law enforcers. This finding fits with Matza's (1964) theory of drift in which he suggests that offenders often find certain types of offending 'easy' to undertake – Matza calls this 'preparation' which, coupled with 'will' and 'neutralization', makes it more likely that an offence will be committed.

MacDonald *et al.* (2001) comment on the importance of locality in circumscribing life chances: the levels of deprivation, crime and drug use in an area can have major repercussions on young people's likelihood of committing crime. Several respondents, more male than female, commented on poverty or negative images within the area in which they lived as being an influence on their propensity to mix with 'the wrong crowd':

> Most people in [local area] have got nothing and we haven't till we get something. [*MB: So do you think if you'd been born and brought up in [affluent area] you'd be the same as you are now?*] No. I'd be different, I'd be a totally different person. I think it's maybe the area.
>
> (Vic, 23)

> It was just pure boredom about here, living about here. There's nothing here. They were only starting to bring little things into this place, but there wasn't anything here years ago ... Oh, don't get me wrong, like, it was all down to money and that. I never had much money and things like that, so we couldn't go everywhere, know what I mean ... My mum done enough for us, aye, but never had all the money in the world to go to the cinema, go places every night, things like that, play golf, whatever. Play football, that's all we ever played, football in the square, whatever.
>
> (Frank, 22)

Whilst school exclusion, truancy and a disaffection with the school curriculum suggested a lack of cultural capital in terms of qualifications or skills development, rebelling against schooling also enhanced their status, and hence symbolic capital, within the friendship group. Some spoke of truancy as also offering a strategy towards having the time to shoplift:

> ... you've got that many orders, you're skidging school [truanting] to go in and get [the] stuff.
>
> (Bernadette, 23)

Cultural capital can be gained through 'street cred' or being a successful offender, and this will be explored in greater depth in the following chapter. However, in terms of academic achievement, positive cultural capital was mainly gained in childhood through encouragement at school, and some mentioned good relationships with teachers in residential schools which facilitated a greater propensity to study. Two young men spoke highly of their time in residential schools whilst in care:

> They don't treat you like shit. They listen to what you've got to say.
>
> (Frank, 22)

> [It was] different from any other school ... just the attention, seven to a class ... it's brilliant man ... you got treated like, like a young man. Other schools you got treated like an idiot.
>
> (Derek, 21)

The advantages and disadvantages of starting offending

When respondents recalled starting offending, there did not seem to be an association between the different advantages that these young people cited and whether or not they had made a conscious decision to start, although the monetary gain from offending was obviously considered to be an advantage as well as a reason.

Monetary advantages

By far the most commonly cited advantage was money, accounting for over half of all responses, irrespective of whether or not monetary gain had been a *reason* for starting. As Kevin, 23, explained, the advantages of stealing were that: 'You don't have to wait a week to get paid'. Money was needed or wanted not only as a means of gaining status, but also to buy drugs, better clothes or, in the case of the women, items for their house or for their children. Women were more than twice as likely as men to see money as an advantage of starting, partly because of their greater need for drugs but also because conspicuous consumption and body image were part of the female youth culture, notably at a time when sexual relationships were becoming more important to them (Skeggs, 1997). Six women cited money for drugs as an advantage of starting offending, but this was because they felt the need to offend in order to maintain an existing drug habit. However, once they were in the maintenance phase of offending, money for drugs became a more commonly cited advantage, as will be seen in Chapter 5.

For many, having money through offending enabled them 'to keep up with the Joneses'; access to money was a status symbol rather than a necessity, as the following quotations illustrate:

> Just having things that other kids had, you know, that I didn't have. Like simple things, like a bike or something like that. Something that we never had, like.
>
> (Nick, 28)

> Not having to worry about spending your money ... Just to keep in with the crowd.
>
> (Sarah, 27)

> [Shoplifting] gave me confidence. I felt going with somebody else's cheque book and getting all dressed up and going in [to a shop], I could spend what I wanted, they treated me well because they thought I had enough money. They had a different outlook ... It was like a power trip.
>
> (Gillian, 29)

Personal advantages

More men than women cited the personal advantages of the buzz from offending and relieving boredom through offending:

> It stops life being a bore, cannabis, speed and ecstasy does ... and it makes me happy.
>
> (Sam, 23)

> We used to hang about with older people ... it was just boredom, hanging about doing nothing and that. Going out stealing cars and things like that.
>
> (Frank, 22)

Whilst none of the women mentioned such personal factors as *reasons* for starting offending, they were more likely to cite such factors as *advantages* accruing from offending.

Relational advantages

More women than men mentioned the relational advantages of offending, in particular where the young people saw offending as a means of keeping in with or generating a certain circle of friends:

> ... my pals liked me better.
>
> (Avril, 18)

> ... it was like I was buying my friends by doing what I was doing.
>
> (Carol, 29)

One's reputation as an offender – either in gaining money or in being 'hard' – was also a key concern to many of the young people early on in their offending. Finally, five men and two women could think of no advantages of starting offending, but the five men started as a result of alcohol misuse, boredom or as a means of making friends, with no utilitarian motives in mind:

> There was [no advantage], it put me in a worse position.
>
> (Pete, 19)

The two women who could think of no advantages to starting offending suggested that they started as a result of drinking to relieve depression or anger following domestic or childhood abuse.

When respondents spoke of the disadvantages of starting offending, their responses centred predominantly upon the practical consequences in relation to themselves and the relational consequences pertaining to other people. As with the advantages of starting, there did not seem to be an association between types of disadvantages cited and whether or not the young person had drifted into, rather than consciously decided to start offending. However, the women were almost twice as likely to think of practical and relational disadvantages compared with the men, for example, becoming involved in the criminal justice system or alienating one's family and (law-abiding) friends.

Practical disadvantages

The majority of respondents spoke of the practical inconvenience of offending, with 'getting caught' being the main disadvantage of starting offending. Whilst many suggested that they did not think about getting caught at the time that they started and some implied that the children's hearing system[1] would not be a deterrent to them starting offending, they nevertheless suggested in retrospect that involvement in both the children's hearing and criminal justice systems was a major disadvantage to starting offending. This was much more the case for the women than the men, since the former were more aware of the stigma attached to crime. As much feminist theory suggests, women are 'doubly damned', not only in transgressing the legal code, but also in transgressing the 'feminine' code (Brown, 1998). This also had negative implications for their relationships, as noted below.

Relational disadvantages

Both male and female respondents were mostly concerned about upsetting their families by starting to offend, and the women were much more likely than the men to be concerned about getting a bad reputation within the community:

> I let my mum and dad down, I let myself down. Ended up in a lot of trouble, school, police, my mum and dad as well. The whole family was really let down.
>
> (Bernadette, 23)

> Just embarrassing my father because he was on his own with four kids, trying to bring them up, and I'm going out and offending ... he had a phone call at his work saying 'your daughter's lying in [the police station], will you come and get her', and then the school, I wasn't going to school, and the school got the social workers involved.
>
> (Carol, 29)

> I was always getting taken away. I was always like getting in trouble. My mum and my father couldn't trust me. I lost a lot of trust ... Getting the trust at a young age is very important to

anybody. But to myself, I felt that not having the trust was a big disadvantage.

(Owen, 18)

Women, in particular, value their good reputation with others, not least because of their seemingly greater commitment to relationships more generally (Gilligan, 1982; Adler, 1985). Ironically, it was in search of a reputation, within their primary reference group (Bromley, 1993), that many of these young people started offending, and yet they still thought (albeit perhaps retrospectively) that their 'good' reputation might concurrently be damaged within the secondary reference group of wider social networks (including the police and businesses), although more so for the young women. Thus, although their reputation with their friends was more important to them *at this stage in their lives* (the phases of childhood and youth), in retrospect, they suggested that their reputation in the wider community and within the family was equally important. One young woman felt this stigma particularly acutely in relation to a local supermarket, from which she had shoplifted as a child:

The disadvantages of getting into trouble? ... Getting caught, going to court, being barred from, like, the shop. Not being able to go in there. Even when you're with your mum and that, I couldn't go in ... We're still barred from there today.

(Sarah, 27)

Another was concerned by the reaction of the police, which only served to exacerbate her bad reputation within the community:

Getting a bad name with the police. Em, and for the slightest thing I did wrong after that, it was just a case of, right, cuff cuff, away to the cell for the slightest thing I did wrong. Walking down the street ... getting sneered at and scoffed at by the police and things like that ... once they know who you are ... they'll sneer at you and scoff at you and, you know, make comments about court the next week ...

(Karen, 28)

Friends and relationships

The peer group is already well documented as integral to a youth lifestyle and as a vehicle towards social identity and status (see, amongst others, Farrington, 1986; Miles *et al.*, 1998; Reiss, 1988). For example, Miles *et al.* (1998: 83) suggest that young people establish 'reference groups' with the implicit aim of having a 'sounding board' for their developing identities. Thornberry and Krohn (1997) suggest that peer groups exert most influence during the adolescent years, partly because adolescents spend more time in group activities with same-age peers and less time with their families or in one-to-one friendships. Greenberg (1979) and Thornberry *et al.* (1991) also highlight the concomitant reduction in parental influence with an increase in the influence of friends. The extension of the transition period between childhood and adulthood (Coles, 1995), and the concurrent dependence on the peer group for longer periods in youth, has also 'increased the vulnerability of teenagers to the expectations and evaluations of their peers' (ibid.: 593). In the longer term, peer groups also play a major role in choice of partner for marriage and procreation (Rutter *et al.*, 1998); thus, peer affiliations could be seen as a testing ground for future relationships of this kind.

Clasen and Brown (1985, quoted in Ungar, 2000: 167) describe 'peer pressure' as being the pressure to do something 'no matter if you personally want to or not'. However, although often not explicitly stated, the inference from the criminological literature on subcultures is that peer *pressure* is a problem only in relation to adverse influences, such as offending or anti-social behaviour. Whereas Glueck and Glueck (1940) dismissed delinquent peer group association stating it was merely a case of 'birds of a feather flock together' (Rutter *et al.*, 1998: 193), Sutherland and Cressey (1978) see peer groups as being the main impetus for the development of delinquent behaviour, but several studies suggest that friends have a minimal impact on offending behaviour (e.g. Kandel, 1978; Rowe *et al.*, 1994). Others suggest that being part of a delinquent peer group encourages offending and having non-delinquent friends encourages desistance (e.g. Farrington, 1986; Loeber *et al.*, 1991; Jamieson *et al.*, 1999). Rutter *et al.* (1998) conclude that:

> ... there are strong selection effects by which antisocial individuals tend to choose friends who are similarly antisocial

but, even when this tendency is taken into account, the findings show that the characteristics of the peer group exert an influence on the individual's likelihood of persisting or desisting with their antisocial activities.

(ibid.: 195–6)

Becker (1963) equated the importance of friendships with an interactionist approach, whether such interactions are deviance-related or not. In suggesting that interaction with friends offered a valuable source of personal identity in the transition to adulthood, Becker suggests that young deviants value their relationships with offending peers in much the same way as conforming young people value their relationships with law-abiding peers, as a means of reasserting their own identities. Recent qualitative research suggests that young people develop their own friendships based not on offending *per se, but* on equality, intimacy and mutual understanding, positive factors which, to many young people, tend not to be present in their relationships with adults (Waiton, 2001). Holroyd (2002: 12) supports the contention by Ungar (2000) that: 'one of the primary advantages of the peer group is that it allows for both the construction of a collective identity and the development of personal power and agency', irrespective of whether or not that peer group is delinquent. Ungar (2000) concludes that young people move from a feeling of disempowerment and worthlessness within the family to a feeling of confidence and wellbeing within the peer group. Many young people cite protection and sociability as reasons for congregating in groups, rather than for power and reputation (Prasad, 2003), prompting Waiton (2001) to argue that 'peer preference' should replace 'peer pressure' in discourses on young people's social networks.

The importance of one's friends or relationships was also integral to the reasons and explanations given for starting as well as stopping offending. These young people were not so much propelled by friends into offending but did so proactively in the company of, or in order to please or help, their friends, partners or siblings. Reasons and influences revolving around friends and relationships rated highly in these respondents' perceptions of why they began offending but there was, nevertheless, an element for many of feeling 'under pressure' to conform. However, as noted above, the blanket expression 'peer group pressure' is misleading since it does not take into account all the nuances and choices of relationship that exist amongst young people. Whilst many studies of criminal behaviour amongst young people cite peers as a major adverse influence, few actually dissect the relevance and importance of the peer group, not least in relation to sources of personal and social power and status.

It is thus argued that peer pressure is therefore not always one-sided or coercive and individual young people are not always social vacuums or necessarily vulnerable within the peer group (Ungar, 2000). Although young people may 'sacrifice personal agency' (Ungar, 2000: 177), this can often be explained as a transitional phase between dependence on family (social control and disempowerment) and independence (autonomy and empowerment). Ungar concludes that associating consensually with peers is 'a consciously employed strategy to enhance personal and social power' (ibid.: 177). To Emler and Reicher (1995), reputations as well as identities have to be established through *visible* activities such as being within a group setting and conforming to group norms, activities which are in contrast to and go against wider social expectations. This requires not only personal agency but also 'strategy' (Bourdieu, 1977).

In this research, three types of agency or strategy emerged which related to other people, namely, propensity to conform (to the friendship group's activities, requests or demands) for *sociability* reasons; propensity to conform for *self-preservation* reasons; and propensity to conform for *personal* reasons. Each of these tendencies is explored below.

Propensity to conform for sociability reasons

It has been suggested that reputations are of as much concern to offenders as they are to law-abiding individuals, in that the former are also keen to promote and sustain a particular kind of external image (Emler and Reicher, 1995). However, the intended recipients of such external images change over time according to need and lifestyle and it could be argued that in childhood the family is the focus of one's reputation; in adolescence the friendship group is; and in adulthood friendships, relationships and the wider community are. Research on childhood interactions with others suggest that friendships have the most influence and impact during adolescence, and particularly on adolescent-limited anti-social behaviour (Rutter *et al.*, 1998; Thornberry and Krohn, 1997). The tendency of young people to congregate in groups is also seen as offering a sense of belonging as well as sociability, especially for young women who suffered parental neglect or abuse as children (Messerschmidt, 1995).

The young people spoke often of not wanting to be 'left out' by their peers and tended therefore to conform to the group's activities, however deviant these may have been:

> I was in the company of other people who were offending. They knew what to do and I just followed their lead and just got involved as well.
>
> (Owen, 18)

> It was just to prove to the older people that I could do it just as well as them.
>
> (Carol, 29)

As noted earlier, there was an element of mimicry or social learning in their desire to conform to the group's activities (Sutherland and Cressey, 1970). However, some respondents on reflection suggested that offending was often more likely to result in one losing rather than gaining friends, although this obviously depended on whether or not their friends were also offending:

> It never got me friends. You always had the same friends. It's really hard to explain.
>
> (David, 20)

> There again, you lost friends as well, at the same time that you gained. You lost one, you gained two.
>
> (Vic, 23)

Propensity to conform for self-preservation reasons

It has been documented that young women (as girlfriends or partners) seem to have one of the most calming and controlling effects on young males who offend (Coffield *et al.*, 1986), but not necessarily vice versa. Jamieson *et al.* (1999) found that for women in particular, having a partner might be more likely to encourage persistence in offending than desistance, if that partner is also an offender. Indeed, if one's attachment to one's spouse is based on threat or compulsion rather than reciprocity, as in an abusive relationship, then the likelihood of persistence in offending is greater (Katz, 2000). Whilst some of the young men felt 'obliged' to offend alongside their peers for sociability reasons, several women felt decidedly under pressure to comply with the offending behaviour of, in particular, their boyfriends for self-preservation reasons. This justification for offending was wholly a female response. MacDonald and Marsh (2005) identified many women in such situations in their study of young people growing up in disadvantaged, high crime communities, where violence from pimps and addiction to heroin locked young women into prostitution.

The young women in my study suggested that their boyfriends used them as accomplices in crime and possibly withheld love, attention or drugs accordingly. The following quotations highlight the fear of violence from boyfriends amongst many of the women:

> ... my boyfriend ... he trained his ex-girlfriend ... I'd get battered, know what I mean, and I'd want the drugs ... He only gave me a wee hit [shot of heroin] and say 'go away and steal' and he wouldn't give me another hit until I had stolen a lot, know what I mean.
>
> (Laura, 27)

> I just knew I needed to [offend] ... If I didn't, I knew I would get battered from him at the end of the night ... He'd hit me, fling cups at my head and ashtrays and slap me if I didn't get the things I was told to get. So he was making money off me but giving me the speed that he was dealing. After being at the court and that, I knew I still had to go and steal.
>
> (Nina, 23)

It has been suggested (e.g. Campbell, 1981; Gilligan, 1982) that young women are more likely than young men to seek personal relationships as a means of self-identity. Certainly, the young women in this study tended to start offending later than the young men and their age and increased maturity alone may have explained the greater likelihood that these young women would be in sexual relationships when they started offending. Where drug abuse was already problematic for one or both parties in the relationship (as was the case for many of the women in this sample), the tendency for these women to offend with (or on behalf of) their partners became even more likely.

Propensity to conform for personal reasons:

Emler and Reicher (1995) suggest that like-minded peers offer young people self-esteem and status, not least when children who offend tend not to be liked by children who do not (Parker and Asher, 1987). However, Emler and Reicher question the logic that young people with low self-esteem will resort to delinquent activity purely as a means of boosting their self-esteem. If one supports the view that young people look to each other for support and encouragement in the transition to adulthood rather than being concerned about what 'adults' think of them, then the association between deviance and self-esteem would make sense: young people gain greater self-esteem from being with friends who collude in their behaviour and actions, even if that behaviour happens to be deviant. Barry (2001a), amongst others, found that young people consider friends to be more important than their families and other adults, in terms of being able to confide in them during the teenage years in particular.

Both Derek's and Pete's narratives earlier in this chapter exemplified the need of many to conform to peers for personal reasons – in order to gain and maintain friendships in childhood. Whilst the majority of the sample felt their friendships were supportive and equal in this respect, there were several, including Derek and Pete, who felt they had to 'work at' friendships through offending, as highlighted in the following quotation from Pete:

> A lot of folk looked at me differently once they'd heard that I'd been caught for something. They were like "wow, what's going on" and that.
>
> (Pete, 19)

Reputation was also an important personal aspect in starting offending, because these young people's reputations as offenders gave them power and self-identity:

> When I was selling, when I was dealing [I was proud of my reputation] because you feel as if you're powerful because all these people come to you and they're trying to get, like, a tenner bag for a fiver ... sometimes you feel shite knocking them back, especially if it's a pal, but you do feel powerful.
>
> (Bernadette, 23)

Conclusions

It is within the school environment that children increasingly relate to other children rather than family members for leisure activities, identity and friendship. Nevertheless, since all children, by dint of their age as well as their size, live in a relatively powerless and protected environment, not least within the confines of educational institutions, much of their collective activity involves pushing the boundaries of that environment in ways that may be considered anti-social (Morrow, 2001), leading in many cases to a breaking of societal norms as well as laws. Not only can starting to offend allow certain children a degree of *social* autonomy, prestige and power, it can also offer them added *personal* and *practical* benefits, such as extra money for consumer goods, an ability to relieve boredom or a greater feeling of self or social identity and worth. For working-class children, many of the norms and values of mainstream society often elude them through conventional means, thus they may resort to unorthodox means of gaining success, money, capital or social identity.

Four-fifths of the study sample started offending as children, between the ages of 8 and 15 inclusive. For the one-fifth who started offending after the age of 16 their reasons and influences were more practical and expedient. However, the majority suggested that offending gave them much needed friendships in childhood as well as cultural goods. It should be borne in mind that these young people came almost exclusively from disadvantaged backgrounds that distinguished them in two ways. They were more likely to be disadvantaged in terms of family cohesion and self-identity and they were also more likely to be disadvantaged in terms of access to the wider cultural status symbols often considered important in developing social identity (Miles, 2000).

Offending was a means of gaining attention from friends, partners or family members, whether rationally chosen or not, and may also have given them the money to accumulate capital and ensuing status. The economic capital they gained was seen as useful in acquiring items which brought them social acceptance and status amongst their peers – such as designer clothes, alcohol, drugs, cigarettes and make-up, all of which were seen as symbols of getting older and becoming adult. The economic capital accruing from successful offending, as highlighted in their stated advantages of starting offending, gave them increased status and reputation with their peers. The expression 'buying one's friends' further epitomizes the duality of these monetary and relational aspects.

Creating and sustaining a reputation amongst one's friends seemed to be a key factor in these young people's propensity to start offending, but equally, the damage done by offending to their reputations within the local community was also cited as a disadvantage to starting offending, notably for the women. This ambivalence was a constant dilemma for these young people as they moved through the three stages of offending, as will be seen from this and the following two chapters. According to Bromley (1993), a bad reputation can cause anxiety and guilt whereas a good one can bring self-worth and security. He also notes that reputations that are deliberately cultivated, as evidenced by many of the quotations in this book, are more vulnerable to change.

In terms of gender differences in starting offending, the women tended to cite relational reasons (for attention or friendships) as the main influence in their starting offending, whereas the men tended to cite practical or personal factors. The young women started offending later generally than the young men and cited reasons and influences more associated with their older age or broader life experience. Whilst both men and women saw the financial benefits accruing from starting offending within this sample, the young men cited general monetary gain and excitement with friends as a major factor in starting offending whilst the young women cited the need to pay for drugs or more relational or personal factors to do with relationships, past and present. This finding runs counter to a study undertaken by Miles *et al.* (1998) which suggested that young women placed greater emphasis on consumer goods than young men, in terms of gaining confidence and status from feeling and looking stylish. Equally, this finding runs counter to Pudney's (2002) study where young men are generally more likely to be at risk from drug use than young women and therefore need to offend in order to purchase drugs. This anomaly may have resulted from the fact that some of the women already had experience of drugs and were more likely to start offending *out of necessity* to gain money for drugs rather than for consumables *per se*. The men were perhaps young enough not to be dependent on, or lured by, drugs at that early stage in their offending histories. However, the women were also more affected by current or childhood abuse and the resultant strain and stress was likely to exacerbate their drug use.

There were various personal, monetary, practical and relational factors cited by these young people in relation to their reasons for, and influences, advantages and disadvantages in, starting offending. Nevertheless, it is concluded that starting offending revolved predominantly around the need for identity and status within their immediate circle of friends as they moved from relative dependence on the family to the more autonomous milieu of the friendship group. The women were more than twice as likely as the men to see the advantages of starting offending. Indeed, their calculation of the monetary gain in starting offending makes the fact that they eventually stop offending all the more incongruent, given that they apparently stopped more easily than the men. Likewise, given that the men could see few advantages in starting offending, it is perhaps surprising that they carried on with such activity for as long as they did. As will be seen in Chapter 5, however, the balance of advantages to disadvantages changes as dramatically as the reasons change, once one moves through the phase of starting to that of maintaining offending behaviour.

Chapter 5

Coming to terms with offending

... once you start doing it, I mean it just starts escalating, doesn't it ... . One minute you'll be shoplifting out a shop and you'll be running out, your heart will be pounding and you'll be like 'oh I done it, I done it, I done it', you know ... And I mean, it's only a sweety or something but then the next day it's like two sweeties and then 'oh I bet you can't get that game'. And you're like 'Oh, I'll have that'. And then it starts doesn't it ... . it just goes whoosh. Nobody can control it.

(Nick, 28)

Introduction

The findings in this and the previous chapter demonstrate how different the two phases of onset and maintenance are for those directly involved in offending. Whilst the previous chapter focused on the first phase, onset, this chapter explores young people's perceptions and experiences of maintaining offending behaviour. Given that many of these young people were actively engaged in offending over a period of between 10 and 20 years, during which they passed through the phases of youth transition, this separation of the two phases of offending seems all the more justified. This chapter also examines the reasons for continuing to offend for those 10 men and 2 women who reported that they had not stopped offending at the time of interview.

The rationale for continuing to offend

Offending in the maintenance phase was seen by the majority of the young people as a necessary means of funding and maintaining a certain lifestyle rather than something that they chose to do in order to make or sustain friendships as in the onset phase. Throughout the sample, offending behaviour either escalated or remained high in youth, often because such behaviour became entrenched or 'routine', an addiction to drugs took over or because it was successful in giving them capital through status, consumables or financial independence. The symbolic capital gained by successful offending increasingly came from having 'customers', but as the necessity to offend 'to order' took over, offending often became a solitary activity, almost a business, thus negating the original emphasis on sociability and fun described in the previous chapter.

Whilst monetary gain for consumer goods as opposed to drugs was a key factor in starting offending, only a minority of respondents suggested it as a valid reason for continuing to offend, even though consumerism is increasingly seen as a crucial factor influencing the lifestyles and choices of young people (Ferrell, 1995; Miles, 2000). However, as was seen in the previous chapter, consumerism amongst young people is often closely aligned with social status – wearing the 'right brand' of trainers is likely to enhance one's popularity with existing or potential friends (Miles *et al.*, 1998; Morrow, 2001). Thus, the consumption potential of offending was more related to its social and symbolic impact rather than to economic gain *per se*. Morrow (2001), for example, highlights the interrelationship between monetary gain and status in her study of 12–15-year-olds, where the young people equated designer clothes with a guarantee against marginalization within the peer group setting. As one young man in my study explained:

> If you come in with a cheaper pair of trainers than everybody else, then you're just gonna get slagged for it.
>
> (David, 20)

The social and symbolic impact of consumption seemed more important in the onset phase than in the maintenance phase, partly because in the latter phase sociability was replaced by routine and social status by personal necessity. Vic, for example, came to realize in the maintenance phase that the kudos from being a successful offender was often eroded by periods of incarceration. However, he persevered in that behaviour mainly for the economic capital accruing.

Vic, 23, persister

Vic's main reason for continuing to offend in youth was that theft and selling stolen goods was profitable and made him feel a part of his network of friends, hence giving him all four sources of capital. At 15 or 16, he suggested his offending shifted from being a source of social capital to being mainly one of economic capital. His offending then reduced in his late teens because he was *'sick of'* always being imprisoned: *'In 7 years, I've been home a matter of 18 months – one year and a half outside, since I turned 16 ... As soon as I get out, I'm away doing it again.'* Prison seemed like *'home from home'* to him, but did not outweigh the benefits of the economic capital accruing from offending between periods of incarceration: *'what I can make in 5 minutes, people couldn't make that in a month'*. As he said in relation to the money gained from offending, if he had saved all that he had made through crime: *'[I] would have had plenty of money ... I would have had my own business if I had kept my money'*. Having 'customers' (social and economic capital), being acknowledged for his skills at offending (cultural capital) and the resultant reputation amongst his peers (symbolic capital) gave Vic a purpose in life and a sense of achievement, however short-lived his periods of living in the community. Although continuing to offend into his mid-twenties, he was getting tired of it, feeling he had been doing it for too long: *'It's not the same as it used to be – it's like a routine now.'* He also knew he was upsetting his mother by continuing to offend: *'She's the only person I really care for a lot'*, suggesting that offending, however successful, was not a lasting or meaningful source of capital for him.

Many respondents, and more so men than women, suggested, however, that they continued to offend for less sophisticated, more opportunistic or pragmatic reasons than for an improved lifestyle or for consumer goods, with the cost of buying drugs being a major reason. The following quotations sum up the mood of many respondents about the petty but pragmatic nature of their offending:

... well, all the crimes regarding the theft and the stealing and things like that, that was just to get money for drugs. Drug offences were unavoidable due to the fact that I took them ... breach of the peaces and that, that's just idiot, basically being either drunk and shouting and going up the street, or shouting abuse at somebody ... The assaults, that's just problems with other people, getting in the way of things that they shouldn't be getting in the way of. Or saying things about other family members or things that shouldn't really be said, you know. So it was just a way of sorting problems out.

(Martin, 24)

Well, when you're drinking and using solvents and that, you're always going to get up to mischief, and that mischief will be petty, you know. It's not going to be like HB [housebreaking] or it's not going to be shoplifting or anything, unless you're stupid.

(Nick, 28)

To use the concepts of structure and agency (Giddens, 1984), it could be argued that in the face of structural adversity and feelings of disempowerment, many of these young people resorted to individual agency, however unconventional or illegal, to resolve problems that may have been seen by them as of a structural nature. For example, one young man described his reasons for assault, police assault and attempted murder as 'using your fists to solve problems'. Whilst for many offenders, such an approach may seem like 'rational choice', it also reflects *a lack of* choice over how to express their grievances within the wider community. 'Strain' and 'status frustration' (Merton, 1957) may thus result in rebellion – whether this be seen as subcultural or personal – against the status quo.

The nature of offending over time

Respondents were asked why they committed certain types of offence and not others, this question being a means of gauging their reasons and justifications for offending over time. Certainly, shoplifting was the most common offence committed by these respondents because it was seen as 'easy money' (for drugs or other consumables) and less risky compared with, say, housebreaking or fraud. However, such offending tended to start off with smaller items but led on to more risky and serious activity as both the opening quotation to this chapter and the quotation below make clear:

> ... the shoplifting, that was mostly for drugs. I used to shoplift for myself to begin with, you know, just wee things for myself, then I started doing it as a business where I was shoplifting every day to make money.
>
> (Harry, 26)

Whilst many saw shoplifting initially as the most convenient offence to commit, some respondents were adamant that they would never, mainly for moral reasons, become involved in other forms of theft, such as housebreaking, however desperate they were for money. Others tried to justify their broader definition of offending according to a sense of social justice rather than personal morality:

> I disagree with [the law defining as criminal] ... when you're homeless and you don't have nothing at all, and like when you're sleeping outside and when you're a lassie and you're scared and you break into cars for somewhere to sleep, or you do something because you're petrified ... or if I stole like a sandwich out of a shop. I know that's still stealing ... there's things that you have to do to survive.
>
> (Nina, 23)

> I don't thieve from houses ... Just anywhere apart from houses ... Just totally invading somebody's privacy, it's just wrong ... it's just what I expect of myself.
>
> (Charlie, 21)

> ... robbing people and stealing handbags and things? I just don't agree with that ... I hate people who take liberties like that and rob old women. I just think that's disgusting. It wasn't every day that I had smack to smoke, you know what I mean, and there was plenty of days when I sat and rattled [had withdrawal symptoms] and rattled and rattled for days and days ... people that can't rattle for one day go out and rob an old woman ... I just couldn't do it.
>
> (Bernadette, 23)

Much of this rationalization for choice of offence type was moralistic, although Matza (1964) might suggest that this was more a technique of neutralization, a subconscious justification or internalization of necessity, but nevertheless, their choice of offence was often overtly determined more by circumstances or expedience rather than by any moral decision-making process. Several women mentioned fraud as something they started doing latterly in order to survive with a drug habit, as one young woman explained:

> I did credit cards because you can get cash back and it was easier. It was a lot easier than having to go and steal all day. It was much easier.
>
> (Nina, 23)

Equally, many of the sample – notably the women – made conscious decisions *not* to attempt certain offences because they were aware of the practical limitations:

> I probably would have done [fraud] if I had been a better writer. It's just I'm no good with signatures.
>
> (Cathy, 23)

> I done that when I was about 7 or 8, shoplifting. I always gave myself away. I would take a red neck all the time. I was never good at shoplifting … And my ears used to go red and everything, and I always gave myself away.
>
> (Vicky, 27)

> I'm no into [car theft]. I can't drive. I wouldn't do that. I wouldn't steal a car if you can't drive. You could run someone over. I've no really been into driving cars anyway.
>
> (Derek, 21)

Drugs and alcohol

Substance misuse and crime have tended to show a close association that cannot be put down to chance alone. Whilst Rutter *et al.* (1998) and Pudney (2002) suggest there is uncertainty as to whether drug and alcohol use predispose individual users to crime or vice versa, the data from my research suggest a negative association. In a study conducted by Flood-Page and her colleagues, the peak age of drug use for both sexes was between 18 and 21 and harder drugs such as heroin and crack cocaine tended to be associated with more serious or persistent offending than softer drugs such as cannabis (Flood-Page *et al.*, 2000). Flood-Page and her colleagues also suggest that drug use is 'the most predictive factor in regard to offending' for 12–30-year-old men in particular (ibid.: 56).

Whilst the majority of young people who start out experimenting with drugs do so for sociability or excitement in the initial stages, addiction to drugs or alcohol is becoming an increasing problem for young people as they enter their late teens (Harnett *et al.*, 2000; Taylor, 2000). However, many women also experiment with drugs as a means of coping with past victimization – for example, girls are more likely than boys to be a victim of child sexual abuse and to have subsequent problems of depression, anger and fear (Chesney-Lind, 1997; Katz, 2000). Whilst for many of the women in the sample, drugs were seen as an important medium whereby a (potentially) loving or caring relationship could be fostered with someone of the opposite sex (many offended to help sustain first their partner's and then their own drug use), these social bonds were tenuous and often resulted in addiction and subsequent breakdown of the relationship.

Laura, 27, desister

Laura considered that her second boyfriend, whom she met when she was 14 and who was five years older than her, escalated her offending (theft, housebreaking, fraud and assault) and her drug use, even though such a relationship was a crucial source of social and symbolic capital to her at the time: *'I never saw the money, he always kept the money. He just kept me going on my drugs and bought what I needed.'* As described in Chapter 4, Laura tended to conform to her boyfriend's demands for self-preservation reasons, because she was subjected to physical abuse from him throughout their relationship. However, when Laura left him at the age of 24, she was prescribed alternative medication, having nearly died in hospital through a drug overdose and pneumonia. This was a major turning point for Laura as she was in hospital for five months, which gave her the time and space – and without drugs, the mental capacity – to reassess her situation. She also realized at this point that she could have lost her children (or they could have lost her) through her drug-taking, thus denying her a crucial source of social and symbolic capital: *'I just didn't want to hurt them anymore. I knew I had hurt them enough.'*

Equally, social bonds with non-drug using friends and family often became strained as a result of such addictions and many of the women in this sample talked of losing the trust of their family as a result of drug use (Chesney-Lind, 1997; Leibrich, 1993). Prolonged drug use can often result in increased isolation, irritability, depression and paranoia. That isolation may also be exacerbated by young female drug users being paranoid about their deteriorating body image as a result of ill health (Chesney-Lind, 1997).

For the majority of these young people (16/20 men and 18/20 women), drug or alcohol use was seen as the main reason for, or an influence in, their offending in the past. Of those who saw drugs/alcohol as the main reason for their offending, the majority cited them as the main impetus to their *continued* offending. The vast majority of offences relating to theft were to fund alcohol or drug use, rather than for consumables, and this is in contrast to the reasons given for committing theft at the onset phase, which was predominantly for consumables (although, at that stage, more so for the men than the women). To reiterate, this suggests that in the maintenance phase of offending, the need for money to fund an addiction had taken over from the desire for status, sociability and identity.

Pete, 19, desister

Pete's main offences as a younger teenager were theft and shoplifting, offences that he described as *'the ones that were open to me. They were the only ones that I had the bottle to do I suppose, until I got older, until I hit like 16 ... It was just what was easiest'*. His drug use increased as he went through his teens, as did his alcohol intake, and he felt that his offending was mainly a direct consequence of his substance misuse, which itself was mainly a direct consequence of his traumatic upbringing. He said that drugs and alcohol were *'the only way I could cope with things'*. At 17 he became worried about his heroin addiction, a drug he had been using since he was 16, which required him to increase his offending in order to fund his habit. His mother and best friend were apparently instrumental in persuading Pete to stop taking heroin and he came off it with no medical support: *'They said stop now or you're dead. It will kill you ... cold turkey alright, aye, a week and a half locked in my bedroom in my mother's house ... they did me the world of good keeping me away from it and now I've learned to keep myself away from it.'* Apart from coming off heroin, he was also remanded in custody for the first time at the age of 17 and his girlfriend had two miscarriages during the course of their relationship: *'Reality bit me very hard on the backside ... I realized, you know, what was going on. What am I doing here, you know. I'm in a very big hole.'*

Davies (2003b) suggests that shoplifting and dealing in drugs are the preferred means of funding a drug habit. Drug dealing (as opposed to possession) in this sample was undertaken almost exclusively to fund a drug habit, with more women (8/20) than men (4/20) suggesting they had been involved in drug dealing. Drug dealing was not for monetary gain as such, but rather as a means of maintaining a certain level of drug use, as one young woman explained:

Everybody thinks that you make money when you're dealing. You don't. Although you've got money, it's for your next batch. You can't spend it ... see when you're drug dealing, it's really so that you've always, always got drugs to smoke, do you know what I mean? It's never, I mean, although there's always money there, you can't spend it ... believe it or not, I actually got into a lot of debt when I was dealing because although I always, always had money, it wasn't mine to spend. So I got into a lot of debt and it took me a lot of time to pay that debt off.

(Bernadette, 23)

In that respect, several women put their offending (for money) down to drug debts, which had to be paid off over and above maintaining their drug habit. This same female respondent suggested that she preferred dealing, however, to shoplifting because it was easier:

> There was no need [to shoplift]. [*MB: Because the dealing covered all the money you needed?*] Aye. [*MB: And that was easier than shoplifting was it?*] Aye. Definitely ... people would just come to my door and I was serving them through the letterbox. I didn't even have to open my door.
>
> (Bernadette, 23)

Often the need to feed a drug addiction resulted in one's offending escalating, becoming more solitary and as some respondents implied, increasingly seeming like 'a vicious circle'. For 29 young people (11 young men and 18 young women) who were taking drugs or alcohol, substance misuse was seen to become problematic in the maintenance phase and had increased their propensity to offend.

Yvonne, 25, desister

Although Yvonne drifted into offending through friends, she said she latterly got a name for herself as an offender and her peers expected her to act in a certain way. *'The thing is I'm not hard. When I look back, I'm not, I was just a bully. It was 'cos someone else wanted me to do it. I was scared of the older lassies. I was better off battering this other lassie than getting a kicking from the older lassies.'* She liked her reputation at the time, even though she thought she was being used, but at least she had a purpose, and this reputation gave her increased social and symbolic capital. Most of Yvonne's later offending (assault and breach of the peace) was drink-related; she never got into drugs so this was not a problem for her. Even if she was short of money she would never have committed theft: *'I didn't have the balls basically ... I'm not really that way inclined.'* She suggested that if she had not drunk alcohol, she would never have started offending, unless someone really *'got on my nerves'*, but her reputation with the police and the local community latterly made breaking her cycle of offending more difficult, irrespective of the social and symbolic capital accruing: ' ... *being drunk ... gives you more balls ... I knew that I could fight. I knew that I could hold my own'*. Yvonne married and had a daughter when she was 20, and suffered depression as a result of being rejected by her mother in particular, who had recently been diagnosed with cancer, coupled with the death of her sister (who had been a vital source of social capital to Yvonne in her teens) and the latent reaction of an attempted rape when she was 13. Because of her drinking, she gave her daughter to her husband to look after, thus losing a major source of social and symbolic capital at that time: *'I couldn't take to being a mum. I was still carrying on ... getting drunk. I gave [daughter] to her dad 'cos I was getting into trouble, I had all idiots in my house. Then I was getting her at the weekends .... . I felt she needed a mummy which I couldn't really be.'*

There was a noticeable shift in the reasons for offending if the individual became addicted to a substance and needed money to fund their usage:

> I was getting addicted to speed. When I was 16 years old, I was on an ounce a day, which is £80 so I had to steal to get my habit.
>
> (Nina, 23)

Such problem use was almost exclusively related to drugs (8 young men and 16 young women) as opposed to alcohol (3 young men and 2 young women):

> I didn't realize it was killing me. I didn't think there was anything wrong with me but it got to a point every day you wake up, you do the same thing, you get up, you've the clothes on you had on from the night before, you get up, you find where you're going to get money from, you'd walk for miles and miles, you'd climb a mountain for a tenner at the top of it and you'd walk back down it again and buy yourself a bag [of heroin]. You wouldn't

eat. The only thing you would eat was chocolate. If you never had money for chocolate ... you'd steal a bar of chocolate to keep your sugar level up.

(Diane, 21)

Taylor (1993) has suggested that shoplifting by women for drugs, for example, had to be carefully planned and methodically carried out, not only to ensure adequate monetary returns to feed a habit but also to ensure that the women were not caught. Offending, if successful in terms of monetary gain, was increasingly seen as a business or a necessary way of life which required skill as well as planning:

As my face got known for shoplifting, I stopped that and went into house breaking ... I went on to fraud, credit card fraud ... I was making about £300 to £400 a day and it was just going on purely drugs ... I was a prostitute and using credit cards to go buy clothes to work in.

(Vicky, 27)

Whilst drugs and alcohol were seen as a problem in the past for the majority of this sample, only three men suggested that drugs or alcohol were still a problem for them now, and all three were still offending. None of the women suggested that they had a problem with illegal drugs or with alcohol now, although several felt dependent on methadone, which they considered a problem, health-wise. Four men and six women suggested that although drugs/alcohol had been a problem for them in the past, they now no longer used them and a further five men and 11 women suggested that their use of such substances was now controlled. One man and eight women mentioned that they were currently on a methadone prescription.

When these young women spoke of trying to stop offending, the factor they identified as being most likely to enable them to do this was to address their drug habit, after which offending would cease to be a necessity for them. However, giving up drugs was not easy, given their addiction, their circumstances and their need for support:

It was actually on a Sunday. I can remember it quite clearly. It was the day after my older brother's birthday. I'd walked up ...

to my mum's, went in and I begged my mum to help ... get me in ... like rehab and things like that.

(Diane, 21)

Methadone calms you down and makes me go to sleep and relax, but it's sore to come off it but I want off it. I don't want to be on it. I want babies and a normal life. That's what I want. It's all I've ever wanted.

(Nina, 23)

I was in my bed for four weeks. [My boyfriend] used to have to lift us out the bed to put us into a bath because I was that slow but I got through it. I fought it. I'm really glad now that I did, really glad.

(Sarah, 27)

The impetus to continuing offending

The 12 respondents who considered that they were still offending (10 men and 2 women, all aged between 19 and 26 at the time of interview) were asked why they had continued offending for the period of time that they had to date. The remainder of this chapter focuses on the responses given by these 12 persisters. Given that there were only 12, and all but one of these considered they were offending on a reduced basis, these responses should be viewed with caution. Nevertheless, the data do demonstrate a stark difference between reasons for and advantages/disadvantages of starting offending and those related to continuing to offend.

Throughout the sample, offending behaviour either escalated or remained high in youth, often because such behaviour became entrenched or 'routine', an addiction to drugs took over or because it was successful in giving them capital through status, consumables or financial independence. Very few of these respondents at the time of interview had had periods of non-offending during their offending histories, thus questioning the extent of 'drift' between freedom and constraint over prolonged periods of time (Matza, 1964). Only six respondents (3 men and 3 women) noted that they had stopped offending previously (in 5 of the 6 cases only once) but then had renewed offending soon thereafter. Events which triggered this temporary cessation of offending (which usually lasted under a year) included being imprisoned (2 men), having a temporary job (1 man) and being pregnant (3 women). As will be seen in the following chapter, the majority of desisters in this sample suggested that they made an active decision to stop offending, and in the majority of these cases, this decision was adhered to. Therefore, Matza's theory of 'drift' – at least as far as this sample is concerned – tends only to apply to the short term (i.e. drifting in and out of offending on a daily/weekly basis) rather than to the longer-term (stopping offending for months/years and then starting again), and indeed this seems to be the case for 'adolescent limited' offenders more generally (Moffitt, 1997).

The main reasons given for continuing to offend were predominantly factors seen as being beyond the control of these young people, for example 'force of habit', mentioned by two male respondents, or having a reputation to uphold, also mentioned by two male respondents:

> It's just inside us and I can't get out of it ... I'm used to doing it.
>
> (Vic, 23)

Sam, aged 23, suggested that offending was now a way of life that he couldn't control: 'a habit, like an addiction'. Equally, some came to expect, even to depend on, a certain level of income:

> [I'm] used to having things ... Used to having everything ... The money and everything that comes with it.
>
> (Cathy, 23)

Several respondents commented on the habitual, mundane and almost boring nature of offending over time. This contrasting attitude to offending in the maintenance phase compared with that in the onset phase highlights the need to examine all three phases of offending as a changing process over time. Whilst many of the desistance theorists acknowledge the negative attitude to offending of those in the process of stopping, little research has been done on such negativity in the maintenance phase, which can seriously undermine many theories of offending behaviour, not least those (notably from cultural criminologists) that highlight the excitement generated by offending. For example, this negative and mundane view of offending amongst those young people who were straddling the maintenance and desistance phases is highlighted in a study of female offenders undertaken by Sommers *et al.* (1994), but equally applies to most studies of desistance irrespective of gender composition (e.g. Maruna, 2001; Shover, 1996):

> Over time, the women in the study became … further alienated, both socially and psychologically, from conventional life. The women's lives became bereft of conventional involvements, obligations, and responsibilities. The excitement … that may have characterized their early criminal career phase gave way to a much more grave daily existence.
>
> (Sommers *et al.*, 1994: 137)

However, despite the 'chore' involved, where such offending was seen as an essential activity by the young people in my study, it tended to take on a momentum of its own and could be accommodated with little effort. It could be argued that this 'force of habit' has wider connotations for studies of desistance, in that the status quo (of offending) may be more secure and preferable to desistance which may require a proactive change in lifestyle or peer group. The need to uphold a reputation could also be seen as wanting to maintain the status quo amongst existing friends as a 'face-saving' mechanism, rather than giving up what is known for something that is uncertain:

> I think it was because nobody knew me … I felt as if I had to make a name for myself.
>
> (Martin, 24)

> Just reputation … Just impress people like – aye, me and my friends will go to other pubs, but there will be still people there that will go 'I've heard you're off your heid and that'. No, I'm no. This boy said something. 'Are you taking that?' Ken, they kind of look. I've got to do something about it …
>
> (Derek, 21)

Bromley (1993: 11) highlights this need to *maintain* a reputation gained in the past because to do otherwise would draw adverse attention to their seemingly changed persona: 'The autonomy of reputation, as a process distinct from the personality it is supposed to reflect, is the cause of much ambivalence'. For those who continued offending because their 'customers' expected it, this ambivalence was all the more apparent. Many of this sample became solitary offenders as either monetary success or drug addiction took over from the original sociability aspect of offending. Once their offending behaviour became more solitary with the decreased influence of friends and associates, some spoke of an increased feeling of isolation, which was likewise an impetus to reassessing that behaviour, as will be demonstrated in the next chapter.

Other factors cited for continuing to offend were because of homelessness, being a known criminal and therefore being expected by the police to offend, being unable to control one's temper (in this instance, one of the women blamed alcohol for her temper) and because of a need for money, either for survival or to feed a drug habit. Many respondents saw their offending as a vicious circle, exacerbated by drugs or alcohol, because of either needing drugs/alcohol or being under the influence of them at the time of an offence: 'It was rebellion against the system initially – not enough money. Then addiction to drugs took over, and then the need to have money [for drugs]' (Kevin, 23).

> ... see when I was like on the amphetamines and then coming down, I felt like I could get away with it. It's hard to describe ... in a way I do think it was the drugs ... I did feel as if I could get away with a lot.
>
> (Paula, 27)

Whilst friends were cited by both sexes as directly influencing their propensity to start offending, few suggested that friends put direct pressure on them to continue to offend. Derek's explanation for continuing to offend was, however, an exception to the rule in this respect.

Derek, 21, persister

Derek was at a loss to explain why he continued to offend: *'I'm sick of it. You do get sick of it ... I've got to grow up and fucking have kids and, ken what I mean.'* His reputation in the area was such that other people expected him to act in a certain way and he felt the need to respond accordingly: *'I've always been a thug since I was young so, ken, people start talking. It does, it gets to you ... you want to grow up but they're not grown up so you want to show them ... I'm not proud of [my reputation]. In a way I am, I'd rather be what I am now than be a wee choir boy ... I've just done what I've had to do instead of getting bullied ... I could calm down ... I really do want to do it, but it's, I don't know, it's just like people ... other people will go "check him, he's changed, ken. He's a shite bag. Let's get him" ... It's hard if you're a guy from [housing scheme] and that ... they've got nothing to show [who] they are.'* With no obvious alternative sources of capital in youth, other than that gained within his immediate circle of offending acquaintances, the ability to move away from the status quo became all the more difficult for Derek. He was still offending at the time of interview, although on a reduced basis and had recently found part-time labouring work with his father which gave him both economic and symbolic capital: *'When you've got money, you don't need to [offend] ... you've earned it and it feels brilliant. Earning a wage feels brilliant, man.'*

For many like Derek, who persist in offending into their late teens and early twenties, the 'dark side' of social capital can continue to have an adverse impact on their attempts to desist (Webster, 2004, pers. comm.). Many of the sample in youth still seemed to feel under pressure from the adverse influence of others, whether this be bullying or encouragement by friends or the demands of a partner. For young women, in particular, the influence of partners can have a profound adverse effect on their level of drug use and hence offending, as Anna's narrative illustrates.

Anna, 21, persister

Anna became addicted to heroin when she was 18, partly because her then boyfriend (twelve years older than her) was a heroin addict and she had moved with him to a city, hence losing the social capital of her childhood network of friends. She blamed her boyfriend for the fact that she got into harder drugs which resulted in her offending escalating: *'I got forced into it. Basically my boyfriend turned round and said do you love me? I said aye, I love you. He said, if you love me, try this. I said I don't want to. And he said he'd batter me if I didn't … I hated [the prostitution]. I was in tears every time because of him making me do that, but then he used to batter me.'* A year prior to interview, at the age of 20 and following a prison sentence, Anna decided to leave her boyfriend, move back to her home area and to come off drugs, these decisions being partly influenced by renewed contact with her father. She wanted to prove to the social work department that she was capable of looking after her daughter full time, but suggested that she would not get custody for at least five years, thus denying her a strong source of social, cultural and symbolic capital.

The advantages and disadvantages of continuing to offend

The respondents who were still offending were asked what the advantages and disadvantages were of offending now. Half the respondents (5 men and 1 woman) could see no advantages in continuing to offend, with one young man suggesting it had become an addiction and another suggesting it was a futile, almost incomprehensible, activity:

> No advantages … It's just all losses, eh. There's no advantages. It's about time to grow up. I'm … twenty-one and a half. Anybody else that's twenty-one with a bit of head and a bit savvy will grow up. There's no advantages. You just get prison, eh. It's just, it's just daft.
>
> (Derek, 21)

For the others, the main advantage of continuing was that it gave them money, mainly for drugs but the more successful offenders could also afford better possessions. However, it should be borne in mind that the monetary attractions were an offshoot – and advantage – rather than the main reason for these young people continuing to offend. Five respondents (four men and one woman) suggested that the lifestyle or the money were tempting:

> I can get all the best things. I can have as much money as I
> want.
>
> > (Cathy, 23)

> A better lifestyle … You can make loads of money. Plenty money.
> Live like a king.
>
> > (Eric, 21)

As was seen in Chapter 4, few respondents cited the attraction of being able to get drugs or alcohol as an advantage of actually *starting* offending, with only six women citing this as an advantage at the time they started offending (although these young women had started offending specifically to feed a potential or existing drug habit). Once their pattern of offending and perhaps even their drug use was better established, their capacity to acquire drugs through offending for money became easier for many of them:

> … it gets easier and easier and then people find out and they
> start saying to you, get me this, get me that, so you get money
> and it's more money for the weekends … for dope, and then it
> went on to harder and higher stuff, do you know what I mean?
>
> > (Bernadette, 23)

Apart from the monetary value, none of the advantages cited in Chapter 4 for starting offending applied to the same extent in the maintenance phase. No one mentioned attention from peers, the buzz/fun of offending or the relief of boredom as advantages of offending subsequently. As mentioned earlier, theories which stress the excitement and cultural embeddedness of offending, such as those of cultural criminology, cannot readily explain the mundane and negative nature of offending in the maintenance phase. For many, it had become very much a routine activity either necessitated or encouraged by the expectation of money, with few other attractions. Indeed, whilst only six persisters mentioned advantages to continuing to offend (and these were all for economic capital), all twelve persisters cited disadvantages (and these were all practical, relating to the 'hassle' and stigma of offending); indeed, the disadvantages outweighed the advantages by three to one.

The impact of the criminal justice system weighed heavily on the minds of those continuing to offend and was seen as the main practical disadvantage. As Cusson and Pinsonneault (1986) and others have suggested, getting caught, appearing in court and going to jail are uppermost in offenders' minds as they become older. One respondent, who had stopped shoplifting some time ago but continued to be involved in assaults and drug use, summed it up in terms of 'paranoia':

> Martin: ... there's no way I could shoplift any more. I could not do that at all.
> *MB: Why not?*
> Martin: Because the paranoia gets too much and I feel as though there's lots of people around and you can never ever tell which one's watching you.
> *MB: Well, why were you happy to do it five years ago and not any more?*
> Martin: Because I didn't have the paranoia then ... Because I was doing something new and I thought I was good at it and, em, because I thought I was good at it then I kept on doing it. But I was caught for shoplifting in [town] once. That was the last time I can remember stealing out of a shop ... My day's finally come, you know. If they catch me now, they'll catch me later on, you know. You lose your edge basically and you do have an edge.
> *MB: Is that because of age or something else, or responsibilities?*
> Martin: I think there's a bit of both to be honest but although, having said that, I still know people that are 30, 40 and they're still quite happy doing their shoplifting. It's just, I think it's each individual.
>
> (Martin, 24)

This greater calculation of risk and seeming inevitability of being detected were closely associated with the fear of a loss of freedom and being away from family and friends:

> [The disadvantages are] missing your family, your friends, social life, parties, ken, just, just freedom. That's what it all comes down to. That's it basically.
>
> (Derek, 21)

> I'm causing grief. You get time to think in jail ... I've got more of a conscience now. Jail slows you down.
>
> (Len, 26)

I'm sick of the jail, sick of it, I'm too well known by the police.
They stop and question me for no reason and people judge me.

(Sam, 23)

Shover (1996) argues that age brings greater calculation of the
risks involved in offending and with age comes a greater awareness
of the need for social bonds with significant others:

Successful creation of bonds with conventional others and
lines of legitimate activity indisputably is the most important
contingency that causes men to alter or terminate their criminal
careers

(Shover, 1996: 129)

It is argued in this book, however, that it is not age *per se* that
brings a greater calculation of risk – which suggests that age is not
a dissuasive factor in its own right. It is perhaps the process of
becoming an 'adult' with the responsibilities, status and rights of
adulthood (and thus something to lose) that is a strong persuasive
factor. As Greenberg (1979: 591) notes in this regard: 'the costs
of apprehension are different for persons of different ages'. The
risks for these young people in childhood were minimal compared
with the growing number of risks associated with adulthood, as
evidenced by the increasing number of disadvantages and decreasing
number of advantages of offending cited by these respondents over
the three phases of starting, continuing and stopping offending.
Each respondent had different levels of responsibility and status
and, therefore, by inference had varying levels of potential loss from
offending when nearing the adult phase of their lifecycle; hence, the
importance of seeing offending as a process which runs concurrently
with the process of transition.

Aspirations towards desistance

All 12 current offenders seemed determined to stop offending in
the near future, although several thought it likely that they would
continue to use drugs 'recreationally'. This optimism about stopping
offending seems to be common amongst young offenders, who
often seem on the verge of desisting following every incident of
offending. Jamieson *et al.* (1999) have suggested that women are
even more likely than men to suggest that they have started the

process of desistance, often only within days or weeks of their last offence. Given, also, that the process of desistance is a long and uncertain one, with many opportunities for relapse (Matza, 1964; Leibrich, 1993; Maruna, 2001), it is likely that these young people will perhaps find that their intention to stop will be put to the test on many occasions, not least in the near future.

Both women who were currently offending cited their children as a reason for wanting to stop and because of the fear of imprisonment. One of these women found it increasingly difficult to offend in the company of her daughter as the latter grew older:

> When I'm in shops, she says things like 'mummy, you have to pay for that'. A couple of wee things like that ... She kens I shove things in my bag. [*MB: She's never landed you in it?*]. A couple of times just about. That's why I've had to stop taking her. I had to stop taking her because she started opening her mouth.
>
> (Cathy, 23)

Other reasons for wanting to stop, each cited by one respondent, were: wanting to grow up, wanting a house, wanting a job, not having to worry about the police, not being a worry to others and wanting to drive a car legally. Other comments were that offending had damaged their reputation and its ramifications had limited their experience of childhood as a time of innocence:

> I've lost a lot ... . just basically growing up ... I grew up too fast. I don't know. Just places I should never have been.
>
> (Bob, 20)

As with other studies which elicited the views of people regarding offending (see, for example, McIvor and Barry, 1998a), many respondents suggested that they had to help themselves if they were to stop offending. Whilst others could give encouragement and advice, these young people considered that it was ultimately up to the individual to change their attitude or behaviour themselves:

> [I am] the only person that can help. If you want to do something, you'll do it. If you don't want to do something, you won't do it.
>
> (Bob, 20)

The only person that can help another person is themselves ... It's somebody's own mind that's got to think 'right, I've got to stop this'. Nobody else can do it for you.

(Karen, 28)

Six respondents (including one woman) mentioned either reducing or stopping their drug use as being a key to helping them stop offending, since many saw their offending as purely to feed their drug habit. Jamieson *et al.* (1999) also found that stopping taking drugs or being prescribed methadone were strategies which helped young people to stop offending, more so for young people who had been on drugs for a longer period of time. Other factors which were seen as incentives to stopping offending revolved around the social bonds of finding or remaining with a law-abiding partner, continuing to care for their child(ren), getting help from family members or professionals and keeping away from offending peers. Practical incentives included getting a job or other occupation (to bring in money or reduce boredom), being able to settle into a new area or house of their own and having a 'clean slate' in terms of court appearances/charges.

The growing realization of the social, cultural and symbolic capital accruing through having children was a common phenomenon amongst the women, as both Laura and Anna's narratives illustrated above. Economic capital also became increasingly important to these young people as they grew older, with many mentioning money as a reason for continuing to offend or for adapting their offending to maximize the economic gains anticipated. In terms of both economic and cultural capital, some of the sample spoke of developing skills learnt from older peers or from being successful at offending, which increased their likelihood of continuing to offend. Whilst consumption of clothes, leisure, cigarettes and alcohol were important to these young people in youth, many of the sample – most notably the women – increasingly required money to maintain a developing drug habit.

Five male respondents mentioned reverting to, increasing or merely sustaining their use of drugs or drink as a major obstacle to stopping offending. As Bob, 20, explained: 'It's easier to walk away when you're sober'. One woman implied that if she got back together with her ex-boyfriend, she would revert to hard drugs again, and two young men mentioned potential police harassment as a likely obstacle to them remaining trouble-free in the future. The potential adverse influence of friends who were offending was also mentioned by two respondents and the loss of current employment by one respondent. Being imprisoned was mentioned by one man and one woman as being a likely trigger to re-offending, as was getting caught driving without a licence for one young man.

Conclusions

The data presented in this chapter sugest that the men and women diverged in whether they 'chose' to offend in the maintenance phase. The men seemed to think *less* about what they were actually doing in their offending over time (hence being increasingly opportunistic or habitual in that behaviour). The women seemed to think *more* about their behaviour and its consequences over time and continued to offend through necessity, having calculated the consequences. Likewise, the men were more likely to seek continued status from offending whereas the women were more likely to be dependent on drugs and therefore more compelled to commit specific offences in the maintenance phase to fund their habit.

The image amongst one's peers of being a successful offender was important to the men, in particular in the early stages of the maintenance phase, even though such a reputation may have caused them more ambivalence latterly (Bromley, 1993). Although people cannot be seen as responsible for the reputations others attribute to them, they are nevertheless held to account for that reputation being either sustained or abandoned. In addition, in a community where young people – especially young men – have few alternative sources of power or friendship, maintaining a public image, however difficult to uphold, may serve an immediate and pragmatic purpose. Jamieson *et al.* (1999) also suggest that offending temporarily gives the impression of social inclusion in an otherwise exclusionary phase in the lifecycle. However, to uphold and build on one's reputation as an offender in the transition to adulthood often required these young people to focus in on that offending activity and to view their offending more as a business.

The realization of the adverse effects of offending became apparent only when such offending became a 'hassle' and unprofitable, and did not fit easily within these young people's developing habitus as young adults. From a Rational Choice perspective (Cornish and Clarke, 1986), the disadvantages of offending eventually outweighed the advantages, when wider social networks and responsibilities (to these young people and their families) became increasingly valuable to them. They seemed no longer to want the often risk-laden capital accrued in the childhood and early youth phases but wanted to progress to adulthood and new, more conventional forms of capital accumulation.

The number of young people who suggested they were still offending at the time of interview is relatively small (two women and ten men). Six of the ten men and one of the two women had made an active decision to *start* offending, suggesting a greater awareness of the possible advantages of offending, at least early on in their offending. It could also be argued that these 12 young people were more successful at offending and therefore did not want to desist, but this was neither borne out by their accumulated offences listed in the SCRO data nor by their seeming dissatisfaction with their current predicaments. In addition, five of the men and one of the women were currently living with their parent(s), suggesting that such close family contact is not automatically conducive to desistance (although see Graham and Bowling, 1995).

Those who continued to offend cited factors that might help them to stop offending in the future, including coming off drugs, being responsible for themselves or others and wanting to 'settle down'. However, because of their working class backgrounds and limited legal and social status in transition, many of these young people's aspirations could have been blocked by poverty, unemployment, a lack of responsibility and a lack of status within the wider community. For example, Hope suggests that, in the current economic climate, unemployment may result in young men of working age feeling they have no stake in society and thence feeling they have nothing to lose by continuing to offend.

When comparing reasons and advantages or disadvantages of *starting* offending with those of *maintaining* offending, the data support the suggestion brokered in Chapter 2 that these are distinct phases of offending which cannot be justifiably combined in an understanding of youth offending over time. The reasons given for *continuing* offending were rarely synonymous with the reasons for *starting* offending, and it seems that the initial kudos, sociability or excitement gained from offending in the onset phase soon wore off as drug use increased, practical need took over or 'criminal justice system fatigue' set in during the maintenance phase. Their offending seemed to become very much a pragmatic means of sustaining a certain lifestyle or habit in the seeming absence of an alternative and perhaps more legitimate lifestyle, and few were currently satisfied with their situation. As Sommers *et al.* conclude: 'involvement in crime moves offenders beyond the point at which they find it enjoyable to the point at which it is debilitating and anxiety-provoking' (1994: 146). It is, indeed, this 'debilitating' change of attitude over time that creates an important opportunity for desistance to be attempted.

Nevertheless, whilst it seems from the evidence in this chapter that offending became a routine or a chore for many of these current offenders, the following chapter highlights the strength and commitment that the remaining 28 young people developed in stopping offending. Whilst the respondents' opportunities overall for conventional lifestyles were hampered by their status as liminal beings (Turner, 1967, 1969), their optimism about stopping offending came across strongly from their narratives, whatever the potential structural constraints (Jamieson *et al.*, 1999; Rudd and Evans, 1998). It is to the views and perceptions of those who succeeded in stopping offending that this book now turns.

Chapter 6

Desistance: breaking free

The true age of desistance from offending can be determined with certainty only after offenders die.

(Farrington, 1997: 373)

Once you start getting into trouble, it's just really hard to get out of it.

(Charlie, 21)

Introduction

The above quotations highlight the fact that stopping offending, or more importantly, *maintaining* a non-offending lifestyle (Maruna, 2001), can be problematic for both professionals and offenders alike. Yet, the actuality of desisting suggests a greater optimism, with Blumstein and Cohen (1987) suggesting that the vast majority of offenders eventually stop offending in their late twenties. The problem is how. There are two concepts within the desistance literature which need to be borne in mind. One is the concept of desistance as *outcome* (measured predominantly by reconviction data) and the other is the concept of desistance as *process* (gauged predominantly by narrative data). Whilst the research described in this book had the capacity to analyse reconviction data for up to two years following interview, its main intention had always been to seek young people's views about their own offending and what events and triggers precipitated or confirmed their desire or propensity to stop offending. To that extent, this study is more concerned with process than outcome. This chapter focuses on the views and experiences of the 18 young women and 10 young men who stated at interview that they had stopped offending. Of the six case studies illustrated in the previous two chapters, only Yvonne, Pete and Laura were desisters at the time of interview. Their three stories of how they stopped offending are, therefore, the only case studies included here.

Desistance as outcome

As Farrington perhaps rightly suggests in the opening quotation to this chapter, desistance is riddled with empirical ambiguities and rarely is it accurately predicted. From an individual perspective, just as a health-conscious but addicted smoker will give up cigarettes and then return to them again with worrying regularity, so the offender may give up crime for days, weeks, months or years, and then return to it (Maruna, 2001). From a structural perspective, when one dissects the meaning of the word 'offending', the problem is intensified. For example, if speeding, dropping litter, urinating in a public place or smoking cannabis are considered to be crimes, then the vast majority of the population have failed to desist from crime, even though they may not have been officially labelled as offenders in the first place. Equally, certain crimes are tolerated in certain populations or at certain times: tax evasion by an affluent businessman may not be such a concern for the police as credit card fraud by a disadvantaged young person, even though Jamieson et al. (1999: 157) cite figures from Cook (1997) which suggest that tax fraud costs the government almost five times more in lost revenue than social security fraud. Labelling theory in relation to offending suggests that young people, disadvantaged sections of the population and minority ethnic groupings may be discriminated against on the grounds of political targeting of certain offences. Certainly, the respondents in this book, although not representative in terms of minority ethnic groupings, were young and disadvantaged and often talked of feeling discriminated against or targeted by criminal justice agencies in particular.

Self-report data on their own can be unreliable, being affected by poor respondent recall, being dependent upon an open and honest perspective by the respondent and possibly being influenced by the respondent's rapport with the researcher. Equally, reconviction data as a measure of re-offending are often ineffectual, in that they incorporate only a small minority of offences and offenders (since only a small minority of offences are detected and processed by the criminal justice system), and often measure reconviction rates only after a short period of time. However, being able to supplement the self-report data with official data in this sample was reassuring in that it confirmed the relative accuracy of respondent recall, although there were a few anomalies. When compared to the official SCRO data on offending histories compiled between 17 and 31 months following interview, it would seem that the female respondents were perhaps overly optimistic and the men more realistic about their status as desisters.

Although desistance may be difficult to measure exactly, there is strong evidence from reconviction and self-report statistics to support a definite decline, if not cessation, in offending activity in the early twenties. Approximately one-third of the respondents who said they had desisted suggested that they had done so two or more years prior to interview, while 14 of the 18 female respondents compared with 6 of the 10 men suggested at interview that they had stopped offending within the year prior to interview.

The young women were not only more likely to start offending later than the young men but they also tended to desist later (only two men stopped offending in their late twenties, compared to eight women). Farrington (1997) has found that the earlier the age of recruitment into offending, the longer the criminal 'career'. He stresses the importance of the correlation between age and crime, with his study indicating a modal age of onset of 14 and a modal age of desistance of 23, although certain studies have suggested that the age of onset will differ depending on the type of offence (e.g. LeBlanc and Frechette, 1989). In this study, early onset did seem to equate with prolonged offending in the young men, but not so in the young women. Nevertheless, this pattern is inconclusive, not least because of the differing ages of respondents at the time of interview, the short time scale between desistance and interview and the small numbers involved overall.

The impetus to stopping offending

This section explores young people's reasons for and influences in desisting and the advantages and disadvantages of stopping offending. It is based purely on the qualitative, self-report data from the interviews with those young people who said they had stopped offending, irrespective of whether or not these narratives were supported by the SCRO data (although, as mentioned above, the two sets of data were remarkably consistent).

Respondents were asked if they had made an active decision to stop offending, as opposed to 'drifting' out of it (Matza, 1964). This was to gauge whether there were any specific 'triggering events' (Laub et al., 1998) or 'turning points' (Maruna, 2001) which might have convinced these young people to change their attitude or behaviour or whether it was more a gradual process of desistance. Bottoms et al. (2004: 383) support Matza's theory of drift when they suggest that 'people oscillate on ... a continuum, between criminality and conformity ... complete criminality and complete conformity are, for the vast majority, points never likely to be reached'. Seven of the 10 men and 16 of the 18 women said that they had made an active decision to *stop* offending whereas, in stark contrast, the majority of respondents said that they drifted into rather than made an active decision to *start* offending in the onset phase. This further questions Matza's (1964) theory of drift as being able to explain desistance, since making an active decision to desist suggests that neutralization and will are eventually and inexplicably set aside by offenders in favour of adopting a specific attitude and approach to the 'problem' of their offending.

Turning points are not necessarily a cause of desistance *per se* but may merely be concurrent with the timing of a decision to stop offending (Laub *et al.*, 1998; Maruna, 2001). Events may be negative as well as positive, thus creating a 'push' rather than a 'pull' factor in one's decision to desist. Giddens (1979: 124) describes turning points as 'critical situations': 'a set of circumstances which – for whatever reason – radically disrupts accustomed routines of daily life', whilst Sommers *et al.* (1994: 125) describe 'socially disjunctive experiences' as precipitating conscious and often difficult decisions to desist from offending. In their study of women offenders, Sommers *et al.* suggest that they all made an active decision to stop, based more on shock than on specific turning points. Maruna (2001) tends to be sceptical of the value of turning points, not least because they can often condemn one to a life of crime or encourage further offending rather than make one more determined to change:

> [Turning points] serve an important symbolic and psychological function, [but] their value to the understanding of desistance has probably been overstated ... nothing inherent in a situation makes it a turning point. One person's reason for changing their life ... might be another person's reason to escalate offending.
>
> (ibid.: 25)

However, Maruna's sample mainly recounted turning points in their childhood years rather than latterly and fitted more into Maruna's category of 'condemnation script' rather than 'redemption script' (2001: 75). However, several studies suggest that it is more recent attitude change, a more mature or heightened awareness of risk and the increasing likelihood of having something of value which could be lost by offending that impinge significantly on offenders' decisions over time (see, for example, Leibrich, 1993; Shover, 1996).

Nevertheless, if an offender *feels* that s/he has made an active decision to change his/her behaviour because of a so-called turning point, this should not be discarded as insignificant, not least when such turning points appear to be dramatically more important in the decision to stop than to start offending. When asked about significant events or 'turning points' in their lives, the respondents in this study were twice as likely to mention events post-16 as pre-16, but the vast majority of these events were 'push' rather than 'pull' factors, not least for the men:

> That was it. Sat back and said 'fuck this'. Excuse my language.
>
> (Pete, 19)

> I'd been caught for housebreaking ... and from then on, like, I thought 'no, that's it, you know. They know we're at it now. The next one's gonna be worse and the next one's gonna be worse than that, and eventually we're gonna get years for what we do'. So I mean, from then, I thought 'no, this isn't it, like. This is not how we're gonna do it, you know'.
>
> (Nick, 28)

> When I was at court one day and I got the probation, I just sat down on my arse and thought: do you give it up or do you do it, because one day you will get the jail and get the kids took off you and it's not worth it. OK you've not got all the nice clothes you did have, and you've not got the money. I can do without things like that just now. I can focus on getting to ... the point where I can go out and get a job and get another bit of my life done instead of stealing
>
> (Helen, 20)

Of the seven men who made an active decision to stop offending, push factors included receiving too many custodial sentences and the need to address a drug addiction. Of the 16 women who made an active decision to stop, push factors included the need to address a drug addiction, abusive partners, bereavement or ill health within the family and fear of losing their child(ren) into care. Three men cited pull factors, including feeling committed to a partner or child and gaining employment. Only one woman cited a pull factor, namely, feeling committed to her partner. As with the reasons for starting offending cited in Chapter 4, the men's reasons for desistance were more practical and personal, while the women's were more relational, although the differences were less contrasting gender-wise in desistance than in onset.

Trigger events which I have described as 'push' factors require agency on the part of the individual to actually change their lifestyle, but with the help of the trigger event as a form of pressure. All the desisters felt that the decision to stop rested entirely with them, and that no external constraints would get in the way of that decision. However, as will be seen in a later section of this chapter, some respondents tempered their resolve with the hypothetical identification of the 'worst-case scenario' which might in the future result in re-offending.

Sommers *et al.* (1994) suggest that giving up crime requires determination and resolve to completely turn around one's lifestyle. Their sample of women street offenders not only had to cease to associate with past 'friends', and suffer the consequent isolation, but they also had, in the majority of cases, to consciously overcome a drug addiction. For many of the women in my sample, stopping offending also meant stopping drugs and so the major decision was more to do with how and when to stop using drugs:

> I woke up one morning and just said 'no more' and I didn't collect my [methadone] script after that ... My partner could tell you. We were going down [to the surgery] one day and I just went like that 'I can't be bothered with this any more. I don't want to do it any more'. And from that day I stopped.
>
> (Sarah, 27)

> I just woke up one morning. I'd slept on a friend's floor ... and I was ill, I needed heroin and I was in lots of trouble with debts, people after me. And I just phoned my mum up and said 'I've

had enough. Give me one more chance'. She came down and picked me up.

(Gillian, 29).

The men did not apparently reach the level of problem drug use experienced by the women, with only one young man mentioning being placed on a methadone prescription as a result of addiction compared with eight young women. Many of the women who were on methadone suggested that offending became an unnecessary activity once their drug use was controlled and prescribed free of charge, suggesting that offending, once they were addicted to drugs, had only been for the purpose of feeding such a habit:

> ... methadone's harder to come off than heroin but rather than stealing, I'm getting it for free ... I don't have to steal to get money now.
>
> (Nina, 23)

> I'm on a methadone programme ... At first I had to offend, now I don't need to.
>
> (Cathy, 23)

These views are backed up by an evaluation by Eley *et al.* (2002) which noted that drug-using offenders were likely to reduce the amount of money they spent on drugs (from an average of £490 per week to an average of £57 per week) as a result of being placed on a Drug Treatment and Testing Order. Equally, the majority of young people in Eley *et al.*'s study suggested that they were unlikely to re-offend if their drug use was controlled. Likewise, McIvor *et al.* (2004) suggest that drug users are only likely to desist from offending once their illegal drug use has stopped.

Factors influencing desistance

Factors influencing desistance are explored under practical factors (including the 'hassle factors' of loss of control of their lives as a result of offending or detection, health factors, the lack of 'success' in offending and the employment and education implications of having a criminal record); relational factors (pertaining to family, partners, children or friends) and personal factors (for example, wanting a better lifestyle or 'growing up').

Practical factors

Overall, the respondents placed greater emphasis on the practical consequences of offending than on relational or personal factors when explaining why they desisted. The two most commonly cited practical factors for stopping were because of a fear of imprisonment (3/10 men and 8/18 women) and the 'hassle factor' (4/10 men and 4/18 women). Several respondents mentioned the 'hassle' which accompanied offending, most notably continued harassment from the police and impending court cases or outstanding charges, which eventually outweighed the social or material gains from offending. The final crunch was often the risk or fear of getting caught and the resultant loss of freedom or control over their movements:

> I'd just had enough ... I had enough of going around and getting lifted by the police and that. Everything what was happening, I was getting blamed for, even when I was in the jail they were coming [to my house] saying that I had been seen, they said 'we saw your son walking down the street with a telly'. I was in the jail!
>
> (Frank, 22)

> I had just grown up, realized the serious trouble I had been in ... and well, at 20, I had my own house at this point ... At the start, I had all nice stuff in it and then like with the heroin, I had sold it all for £20 at a time. Everything, and then I just thought to myself 'what am I doing here? I've got nothing. I'm in my twenties'. Do you know what I mean? ... and I was 'right, that's enough, time to grow up here' ... the police knew ... it was this house I was dealing in, right, and they were sitting right outside ... the door was going constantly ... that was enough. That was enough after that.
>
> (Bernadette, 23)

The deterrent effect of the police and the criminal justice system was remarkably strong for both the young men and the young women. Whilst they talked of having 'had enough', they were actually referring not so much to the effects of ageing or to lacking energy to continue offending ('burn out'), but to being undermined by the effects of being caught and being subsequently embroiled in the criminal justice system:

... you could get away with it when you're under 15, 16. You can get away with crime and that. But after that, you can't get away ... it's not worth going to all the hassle of being in [jail] ... and like you're in there at New Year and Christmas and that, and all your family are outside and that, opening presents and things like that ... and [you] just get pissed off going in and out of the place.

(Frank, 22)

Maruna (2001: 151) has described the 'burn out' model of desistance as relating to 'defiant rebels [who] eventually lose the youthful spirit and passion required to maintain a deviant lifestyle in the face of repeated failure'. Whilst there is undoubtedly a strong correlational effect between 'burn out' and desistance, Maruna (2001) argues that 'burn out' is not a conclusive explanation for stopping offending, as it can as easily happen to active offenders as well as to desisting offenders. 'Burn out' is what Leibrich (1993) calls a 'dissuasive' factor – one that influences desistance because of its negative implications – whereas it is argued throughout this book that for desistance to be sustainable, the positive impact of 'persuasive' factors is needed in that process, as will be demonstrated in the following chapter.

For the women in this study, health reasons (the potential or actual consequences of an addiction) were more of an incentive to stopping offending than for the men, with five women as opposed to only one man citing health as a reason for desistance. Although health comes under the 'practical' category, these women saw it ultimately in terms of relational factors:

It [heroin addiction] was killing me. I was five and a half stone and it was killing me, and I didn't realize it was killing me.

(Diane, 21)

I near died and like, you know, support machine and everything ... so it gave me a fright ... I thought that was gonna be [my daughter] seeing me for the last time.

(Laura, 27)

Many feminist writers have stressed the importance of body image to young women (see, for example, Chesney-Lind, 1997; Skeggs, 1997) as a means of exerting power in an otherwise restricted market, and indeed several of the women in this sample suggested that people would comment on their deteriorating appearance once they were addicted to drugs, and that this negative public image was a motivating factor in their decision to give up drugs.

The men, on the other hand, were more concerned with pragmatic factors such as employment prospects, the effects of a criminal record and offending becoming less profitable and more risky. These findings are consistent with other studies of gender differences in the desistance literature, where women are more likely to take a moralistic or emotional stance in relation to desistance whereas men are more likely to think or act pragmatically (see, for example, McIvor *et al.*, 2004).

Actually having employment or being on a college course (as opposed to the prospect of such opportunities in the future) were particularly influential factors in encouraging desistance for the men. However, whilst employment is often cited as a key factor in encouraging desistance from offending, 24 of the 28 desisters (8/10 male and 16/18 female respondents) did not have employment but still considered that they had managed to stop offending. Indeed, of the five young people employed at the time of the interview (3 men and 2 women), one young man said that he was still offending. Whilst employment was not given as a *reason* for stopping offending *per se*, it was deemed to be an *influencing* factor cited by the three working men but not by the two working women:

> ... just the job [was an incentive to stop] ... just something to do. The thought of getting up out of your bed and working instead of just sitting about all day.
>
> (Alec, 28)

> I can work for money now. I don't need to steal it.
>
> (Rory, 23)

> Well now I've got a job ... Well I've got something to look forward to. I've got something to look forward to when I get up in the morning.
>
> (Frank, 22)

It has been acknowledged in the literature on offending that the lack of employment opportunities for young people – especially for men – may exacerbate their reliance on offending for status and a relief of boredom (Greenberg, 1979; Cohen, 1955). Child-minding restrictions – or in the case of some of the women in this sample, incapacity to work because of drug addiction – may deter women from seeking employment on a regular basis. Employment generally may thus be seen as more important for men in the transition to adulthood than for women, and research demonstrates a higher correlation between unemployment and offending for young men than for young women (Flood-Page *et al.*, 2000). Several male respondents without employment commented on the fact that it was unlikely they would get a job in the future because of their criminal record or reputation as an offender:

> I was working last year for a week ... it's really because of my reputation as well, you know, with being in jail all the time.
>
> (John, 23)

> ... nobody's gonna accept me ... because of my criminal record.
>
> (Owen, 18)

Nevertheless, it seems that the majority of these respondents considered that they were in the process of desisting if not completely stopped at the time of interview irrespective of their employment status.

Relational factors

Many respondents emphasized the support of significant others in the process of desisting from offending, mainly partners, family members, friends, social workers and other agency workers. Whilst Gilligan (1982) suggests that men have fewer friendships than women as they get older, Shover (1996) in a study of older male ex-offenders nevertheless suggests that the social value of interpersonal relationships for his sample of men (i.e. with friends as well as the wider community) should not be underestimated:

> The extreme importance of interpersonal respect, particularly to men who almost certainly are denied it based on their location in class and moral hierarchies, cannot be minimized.
>
> (Shover, 1996: 106)

Relational factors were marginally more influential for the young women (11/18 women compared with 5/10 men), for example, because of now having responsibility for children, because of the positive impact of a relationship or because of the support from family more generally:

> Reasons for stopping? Well the kids, know what I mean. To try and make a family ... [My daughter] had seen so much ... She hadn't seen the needle or nothing, know what I mean, but kids aren't stupid.
>
> (Laura, 27)

> ... having a son. Once he was born, then I really put the foot down ... Because I had someone else I had to look out for other than myself ... my son, he was too young to look after himself. That's my job.
>
> (Martin, 24)

Whereas social control theories are not conclusive in relation to more structural 'turning points' such as marriage or employment, they are useful in relation to the *people* who were influential in helping these young people stop offending – namely, family, friends and professional workers. It is acknowledged that one's family background and the influence of siblings and peers may well have encouraged offending in the past for these young people, as suggested in Chapters 4 and 5. However, as these young people got older they suggested that the negative influences of offending siblings and peers weakened whilst the positive influences of family and 'law-abiding' friends strengthened. This may well have resulted from changes in lifestyle during the transition to adulthood, for example in leaving school and gaining one's own tenancy or finding a job. For the women in particular, having children often resulted in their becoming closer to their own mothers for sharing child care or for financial support (Allatt and Yeandle, 1992; Heidensohn, 1996). Support from immediate family members was particularly helpful to the women. Equally, the women were more likely than the men to be influenced by their own responsibilities towards their partners, family and children:

> I think it's when the social worker said that we've put [my daughter] with prospective adoptive parents and I sort of

freaked out then. It made me more determined to fight for her.

(Sarah, 27)

... with a sentence of 3 years, you're away from everybody that means anything to you. You're away from them all. So it was 18 months I was away from my son. He cried at every single visit ... what I was doing was having – the impact it was having on my family. I mean not the rest of my family, my son really. And I just thought, I can't do this anymore. I can't do that. People say you can't come off drugs ... My son was my staying power. He kept me going. I couldn't do any more to him.

(Theresa, 33)

Certainly for this sample, the social bonds of family and relationships seemed more apparent for the women with partners or children than for the men but it may also have been the case that young women feel more comfortable sharing their emotions and feelings with a researcher than do young men (Oakley, 1981; Phoenix, 1994). The women suggested that they were more determined to stop offending if such offending meant jeopardizing a loving relationship with a non-offending partner. One young woman who became addicted to drugs at 17 because of pressure from her then-boyfriend was now, at the age of 23, on a methadone programme because of encouragement from her current (non-offending) boyfriend, whose threats to leave her if she continued to offend were the major catalyst to her stopping:

My boyfriend would say ... if I stole, he would leave me.

(Nina, 23)

Yvonne, who met her fiancé a year before the interview, stopped offending at that time because of the positive change of circumstances and emotions resulting from this new relationship, as described below.

Yvonne, 25, desister

Yvonne stopped offending aged 24, when she met her fiancé, but this required her relinquishing previous forms of accumulated social and symbolic capital: *'A good man, a different lifestyle away from all the wrong people ... I moved here away from them all and I don't phone them or go and see them or nothing.'* Yvonne wanted to get custody of her daughter again, and had therefore consciously stopped offending so as not to give her ex-husband *'ammunition'* to fight the case. The advantages of not offending were that she had a good relationship and she was free from worry and violence: *'I don't have to be on edge.'* She was also getting more respect from people, as well as gaining self-respect, both sources of symbolic capital. She said she had too much to lose by offending again: for example, the battle for her daughter and her future happiness with her fiancé: *'[My fiancé] brought a really different side out on me. He makes me relaxed, more calmer, and it's like as if I found someone who really cares and actually is interested in me, for who I really was.'*

Knight and West (1975) found that the majority of those who said they had desisted also mentioned that this was an active decision resulting from the breaking of friendship ties with delinquent peers. Indeed, Stewart *et al.* (1994) found that the influence of peers decreased concurrently with offending behaviour as offenders got older. They suggested that 45 per cent of 17-year-olds in their sample were said to have been influenced by peers ('social activity'), whereas only 18 per cent of 23-year-olds were said to have been thus influenced. However, for the young people portrayed in this book, the positive impact of conventional friends seemed to be as much an incentive to stopping offending as the negative impact of offending friends had been an incentive to starting offending. Losing close friendships through crime was sometimes mentioned as a cost:

Em, well you get a lot of friends when you're in one sort of circle but they're not really true friends, and friends that you should have and should keep don't want to know you. So you can lose a fair amount of respect. Although you gain friends, or acquaintances shall we say, you seem to lose a helluva lot of respect from the people that will care about you or people that want to know.

(Martin, 24)

Personal factors

Four women suggested that one of their main reasons for stopping offending was because they wanted a 'normal' or better life, the chance to conform and to 'settle down'. 'Normal' was defined by one young woman as:

... getting up in the morning, doing my housework – although I never done it this morning!... going to the shop, getting the paper, a couple of rolls ... [having] a cup of tea. That's normal for me.

(Bernadette, 23)

I wanted to do something with my life. I wanted to get out of this rut I was in ... carrying on like this and going to court. I was only building up a record for myself and it wasn't the place I wanted to be. I didn't want to be in this situation. I still needed my money, I still needed the clothes, but now I've got to do without that. That's just tough. I've got to live on the money that I'm getting and I'm doing it ... I'll go and get a good job that I want to do and get legal money to go shopping 'cos I'll feel a hundred times better about myself and I've realized that. I've grown up really.

(Helen, 20)

I've got away from all the bad things in life ... I can't be bothered with that ... I'm just getting too old for it. I'm just not wanting to roll about the streets fighting and things like that. It's embarrassing ... I'm not wanting that kind of life anymore, I want to get a house and get settled down.

(Carol, 29)

This increasing pragmatism and disenchantment as they continued offending was closely related to the 'hassle factor' mentioned above, but was also associated with a developing realization that offending was not compatible with their increased need and desire to achieve conventional goals. The vast majority of this sample had identical conventional aspirations to those of young people more generally, namely for a job, a house of their own and a family of their own (Barnardo's, 1996; Barry, 2001b). Thirteen men and thirteen women in this sample mentioned wanting a job, and seven men and ten women cited a house. Seven men and five women mentioned having a settled family life, but only after they had gained stable employment.

Seven men and five women lived with their parent(s) and a further four men and eight women lived alone. Two men and two women classified themselves as homeless and the remaining seven men and five women were cohabiting. Cohabitation and having children seemed to be associated with desistance for this sample, since only two of the 12 respondents with live-in partners suggested they were still offending, whereas 10 of the 28 living alone, with parents or in homeless accommodation said they were still offending. Equally, of the seven men with children, only two were still offending. Both women persisters had children; of these women, one was living in her own tenancy and the other was living with her parents.

The advantages and disadvantages of stopping offending

Respondents who suggested they had stopped offending were also asked what the advantages and disadvantages were of not offending now. Practical factors prevailed as advantages of no longer offending followed by relational factors.

Practical advantages

Four of the ten men and nine of the eighteen women cited the advantage of no longer being a focus of police attention and of no longer being 'paranoid' about being 'hassled' by the police. This was the most important practical advantage of not offending followed by the advantage of not being imprisoned again:

> Well you're not curtain twitching, you're not looking over your shoulder. Look at the grey hair I've got and I'm only 28. Gee whizz, man!
>
> (Nick, 28)

Not having to worry about anything, about the police coming to the door. Nobody can come to me now and say 'you've done this' because I've not done nothing.

(Sarah, 27)

I don't need to keep watching my back. I don't need to keep my eyes open, like when the police pass. I don't need to keep watching and see where they're going. I can just ignore them, you know, and not bother about them.

(Harry, 26)

Particularly the women saw avoidance of imprisonment as an advantage of not offending now, not only because of a fear of being within a prison environment, but also because it would restrict their freedom, their access to their children and their ability to maintain a house of their own:

I don't want to lose my house. I don't want to go to prison. I'm basically getting too old for it. I've got my freedom and I wouldn't like to lose that.

(Carol, 29)

Relational advantages

Improvements in relationships, either with family, partners or their own children, alongside staying out of prison, were equal second in these respondents' lists of advantages of no longer offending. Three men and six women mentioned improved or renewed relationships as advantages to them:

[MB: *What are the advantages of not offending now?*] My son, my job, things like that. I've got my family ... I don't miss it. I'm quite glad that I'm away from it and I'm earning money.

(Frank, 22)

I've got to think about what my family want and what I want. Do I want to go to jail all my life? No. Do I want my mother and father to come and visit me in jail? No. So if I stop offending, they won't come and see me in prison because I won't be there.

(Owen, 18)

Improving one's self-respect and self-worth were seen as advantages of not offending. Certain responses illustrated the need that many of the sample had for the praise and encouragement of family members or non-offending partners or friends. They felt they had achieved a lot by stopping offending and benefited from the positive reaction and encouragement of others. This came across strongly in what they said about not offending now:

> You get respect ... I feel proud because you're not committing offences. You're not letting people down.
>
> (Owen, 18)

> People don't look down their noses at you anymore cos they don't see you as a hooligan. It sort of gives you a bit of respect.
>
> (Martin, 24)

> I don't feel like scum anymore ... [I] feel worth something now. I can make something of myself now. Get on with my life. I want to have babies and I want to get married. I just want all the normal things in life and I feel now that I'm grown up a wee bit and my head's more clearer. I've got a lot of loss of memory with drugs and I've still got a lot of very bad depressions but I've sort of got my family back a wee bit. I don't want to ever lose that, it's so sad.
>
> (Nina, 23)

This developing feeling of interdependence, social identity and empathy amongst the respondents in relation to people in their lives other than their peers is seen as an important factor in aiding desistance, and is discussed further in the following chapter.

Equally, getting older and realizing what one had to lose by offending were important factors influencing desistance. For the women in particular, their reputations were at stake, not least with potential partners. McRobbie (2000) argues that young women are more likely to be concerned about their reputation – as offenders, drug addicts or alcoholics, or concerned about their physical appearance being adversely affected by drugs or alcohol. They are thus, perhaps, more likely to stop or modify their offending accordingly as they get older.

Maturation on its own was thus unlikely to result in capital accumulation – one had to have something to lose, such as a reputation, a partner or an opportunity for legitimate status, before one realized the value of such a potential loss. Employment, a source of legitimate income, responsibility, one's own tenancy and lasting relationships were all factors cited as being of value to these young people in early adulthood. However, as Laura implied, stopping offending also meant losing something of value – the social capital gained from being with fellow drug users or with fellow prison inmates, for example (Sutherland and Cressey, 1978). Thus, the agency required in deciding to stop offending also meant giving up sources of stability, continuity and sociability in childhood and youth.

Laura, 27, desister

A friend of Laura's helped her stop her offending and drug use and this required her relinquishing the social and symbolic capital of her drug-using friends and her boyfriend of some ten years' standing. However, having come off drugs and having left her boyfriend, there was no reason to offend, since her offending latterly was purely to feed her drug habit. She wanted to make a family with her two children and to avoid hurting them any more, and although her ex-boyfriend and others were still trying to dissuade her from going straight, she was adamant she would never return to offending, even though she was sometimes tempted: *'I've had phone calls and that asking if I would sell and all the rest of it, but I'm just not interested ... I think about it right after I've said no. [Laughs] I will say that, I do think about it. I think, I could make money ... but I don't miss it. It's like I'd rather not have the money, know what I mean? I'd rather live off my dole money than have loads of money and have the fear of being lifted and being put in the cells and that.'* The advantage of not offending now was a feeling of self-worth (symbolic capital): *'being free from a damaging relationship ... Being able to lift my head high ... I feel I can lift my head high although people would doubt me. I feel I can walk down the street with my two kids ... considering the state that I was in, know what I mean, I am proud.'* Nevertheless, after three years of being offence-free, she suggested that her reputation as an offender was still apparent: *'everyone would look down on me, they still actually do ... they would still doubt me, know what I mean, and names stick'.* Her determination to remain offence-free was all the more courageous given this lack of social and symbolic capital accruing from a positive reputation in the community. What kept her going was the support of her friend, having her own tenancy and renewing contact with her mother, all crucial sources of capital for her meantime.

Personal advantages

Three men and seven women spoke of the personal gains of not offending in terms of being in control of their lives and having the freedom to be 'normal'. This feeling of being in control, free and 'normal' highlights this sample's overall desire for conventionality and stability in their lives:

> Being free. It's, like, no worry. I don't have to be on edge ... It's good just being free.
>
> (Yvonne, 25)

> ... being able to get a job, then I'll live my life ... I've got a lot more control over what I do. I've got a lot more control where I go, who I speak to, you know.
>
> (Pete, 19)

> It starts to feel good, the fact that you're just a normal, everyday person with a normal job ... and normal money coming in ... I can just do everyday life things that ordinary people do.
>
> (Theresa, 33)

Monetary advantages

Many of the young people expressed a sense of pride of having what one young man described as 'honest money' since stopping offending:

> I'm quite glad that I'm away from [offending] and I'm earning money and supporting my family with honest money.
>
> (Frank, 22)

> You don't need to steal when you're working ... I prefer working.
>
> (Rory, 23)

> Being able to walk into a shop without stealing something ... I go in and buy it ... I like paying for my own things. I like going out shopping and buying clothes.
>
> (Avril, 18)

Economic capital gained from employment rather than offending became a reality for several of the sample, even though such employment may have been casual or short-term. Imprisonment and a criminal record can often deny one access to the economic and symbolic capital of employment. Periods of incarceration often made these respondents feel marginalized from their communities or job opportunities, as did an adverse reputation (as an offender or drug addict) with family or potential employers. State benefits also became an alternative source of income for those aged over 18, and those prescribed methadone found the economic savings considerable. Cultural capital accrued from a renewed interest in educational courses for skills development or career opportunities. Symbolic capital tended to equate with stability in adulthood, through either employment, the status accruing from having responsibilities for oneself or others, being maintained on a methadone programme (and thus not being seen as a 'junkie') or having one's own family or tenancy.

When asked about the potential disadvantages of stopping offending, the vast majority of respondents (8/10 of the young men and 14/18 of the young women) felt that in reality there were no such disadvantages. However, some could think of disadvantages hypothetically – on the whole monetary (3/10 men and 6/18 women) – but stressed that these did not outweigh their determination to remain offence-free in the future.

The lack of money was the most commonly cited disadvantage to not offending, although this was only pertinent to those whose offending had been for financial gain in the past and had been successful in that respect:

Well money. But that doesn't bother me at all. [*MB: So you don't miss the money?*] No. Well, I miss it but [laughs], everybody would!

(Marie, 21)

The clothes I used to get off credit cards, I miss them. Aye ... the money was good. The money was good and I used to get all my clothes and all these designer jackets and all that.

(Vicky, 27)

One woman, however, somewhat resented the fact that she had to pay for such items now rather than shoplift them:

[...] not having any of the things that I could have had. You know, walk into a shop and grab any clothes you wanted. I had as much clothes as I wanted ... and the good make-up, everything. I'm having to buy it now. When you've stole all that time. Like paying £10 for mascara, which I think is ridiculous. I wouldn't dream of paying for that and I actually bought a foundation that was £7. I cringed and I was sitting looking at it and thinking 'I could just lift that in my bag' but I thought 'no'. I bought it, paid for it, and that was it. It's horrible paying for toothpaste and shite.

(Helen, 20)

Craine (1997) also suggests that offending for monetary gain becomes as much a virtue amongst one's peers as it is a vice within the wider society: 'The ability to reap high rewards for the minimum of effort provided status and self-worth within the subcultural milieu' (ibid.: 147). Thus, to give up not only the money, but also the status, requires a great deal of effort on the part of those young people with few alternative means of cultural identity. Nevertheless, it would seem, contrary to cultural criminological theories of offending, that youth culture *per se* does eventually become a secondary source of identity in the desistance phase, when aspirations towards conformity within the parent culture develop – for example, through having a home of one's own or gainful employment. Just as Brake (1985) suggests that young people in a subcultural milieu play off their individual worlds against that of the wider society, so too, in the process of entering an adult-oriented culture, young people may reject previous affinities to a youth-oriented and non-conformist subculture.

However, several respondents implied that they had gradually become used to the changed lifestyle since giving up offending and that it was easier to cope with the disadvantages as time went by:

> ... If you'd asked me that a couple of years ago, I would have said money [was a disadvantage]. Now I'm used to even being on the dole ... at least being able to deal with that, you know. Working sort of round it ... I really did miss that money at first. Now I don't miss it at all really. I've got used to getting by.
>
> (Harry, 26)

For those whose offending was not for material gain, there were no real disadvantages in stopping, apart from losing the excitement. For some, the buzz from offending was sometimes seen as difficult to shake off, as exemplified by the following two quotations from women who had also cited the 'buzz' as an advantage to starting offending:

> When you're shoplifting you get a wee buzz. I sometimes miss that.
>
> (Sarah, 27)

> I miss the buzz, being honest with myself, I suppose I do.
>
> (Vicky, 27)

Sustaining desistance

The respondents who suggested they had stopped offending were asked what might happen in their lives to make them start again in the future. The most common response from the women was that if they were to lose their children for whatever reason (especially if their children were taken into care), this would probably lessen their resolve to remain offence-free. One of the women's strongest influences to stopping offending had been their responsibilities towards their children, and so it is perhaps not surprising that if the children were no longer with their mothers, then the latter may have little reason *not* to offend. Two women also feared that losing a partner or parent would encourage them to start offending again. The majority of the female respondents suggested that they would lose contact with, or the love and trust of, their families (notably their parents, their partners and their children) if they were to re-offend. All these female respondents suggested that it would be drugs or alcohol that they would initially fall back on, but that funding such a habit would eventually lead to offending. Suffering depression or continued physical, emotional or sexual abuse and having a methadone prescription stopped were also cited as obstacles to remaining offence-free:

> If my kids got took away. If they ever got took off us, then I would just go right off the rails and I would be away. That's it.
>
> (Helen, 20)

> If I get struck off my methadone. That is the only thing that would make me start offending, if I was to get cut off ... I'd start back on drugs.
>
> (Marie, 21)

> What would really push us over the edge would be to lose this case [applying for custody of her son]. That's what I'm scared of ... I think I would probably start with the drugs and then it would turn into offending again.
>
> (Sarah, 27)

Many of those who had stopped before in the past suggested that drugs, drug-taking partners or a lack of money or employment were the impetus to them starting again. Certainly, probationers interviewed in a study by Farrall (2002) suggested that drugs and alcohol were the most likely obstacles to remaining offence-free. However, four of the ten men and six of the 18 women suggested that nothing would make them start offending again in the future, as Vicky and Pete emphasise:

> I would never take drugs again. I couldn't put [my daughter's] life in jeopardy ... I'm too strong now, I couldn't ... I couldn't go back down that road. I hit rock bottom and I mean rock bottom and I would never go there for nothing in the world ... Nothing. And I'm positive about that ... I've been through a lot, definitely, I've been through a lot to come off it and it's been really hard ... Oh God, it's been a long struggle to get to where I am.
>
> (Vicky, 27)

Pete, 19, desister

In retrospect, Pete suggested that his offending had never been successful as a means of gaining social, economic or symbolic capital or escaping from childhood traumas. However, three people were particularly influential in helping him latterly: his social worker, his mother and his best friend: *'They sort of made me realize as I grew up that what I was doing was wrong and helped me over the past sort of four or five years'*, and it was this social capital that gave him the impetus to come off drugs and stop offending. Pete suggested he had responsibilities to these people, most notably his mother – *'just to be there in case I'm needed'* – as well as to his current girlfriend, and that if he started offending again: *'[I would lose] my house, my pet, my girlfriend, my mother, all my family, all my friends, everything that I've worked hard for over the last couple of years.'* He was *'proud'* of the fact that he had stopped offending and come off heroin, and was determined to make something of his life in the future, although he was fearful to raise his hopes only to have them dashed again: *'Every time I've set myself a goal, something's gone wrong.'* However, when asked what might happen to make Pete start again in the future, he replied: *'Nothing at all ... not a frigging hope in hell I'm starting offending again. I want to live my life now.'*

Nevertheless, however adamant they appeared that nothing would influence them to start offending again, some of the women tempered this with the need to adequately provide for their children:

> I just couldn't go back. I couldn't. I couldn't go back to that. Start to shoplift to feed the habit. I suppose, we were just talking about it, me and my friend, about two weeks ago – if, say, maybe I had a couple of [children] and things were really tough and I had not a penny, maybe I would say 'right, well I'm going to have to do something here to get money', shoplift or – I mean, I think that's as far as I would go, would be shoplifting. [*MB: To feed the kids?*] Aye, but not to, not to feed the habit.
>
> (Bernadette, 23)

Cornish and Clarke (1986) have identified a certain 'readiness' in offenders to return to crime should the need arise or should circumstances justify it. If asked, individuals will doubtless come up with a 'worst case scenario', as they did in this study as well as in others. Burnett (2003), for example, identified ambivalence and uncertainty amongst her sample of property offenders, where some suggested that if the circumstances suggested they would not be caught, they may be tempted to re-offend, whilst others suggested that sudden hardship or the denial of conventional opportunities might tip the balance in favour of re-offending. However, the majority of the respondents in my study were satisfied with their current lifestyles and optimistic about achieving future goals, such as finding employment, getting their own house and having a settled relationship.

When asked what they had to lose by starting to offend again, the majority cited relational rather than material factors, especially the young women. Leibrich (1993) argues that it is not so much material possessions that deter people from re-offending but the personal values they hold and their changed attitude to those around them. Thirteen women compared to five men cited family or parents and 14 women compared to three men cited their children, although there was more of a gender balance between those who cited their partner or their freedom (through incarceration). Only three men in the total sample felt they had nothing to lose by re-offending, and sadly they also felt that they had nothing of significance in their lives in the first place:

> When I get out [of prison]? I've nothing ... I've no house, no kids, nothing.
>
> (Len, 26)

Recent research on desistance highlights a change of peer group, a sense of direction and 'settling down' as factors associated with desistance (e.g. Graham and Bowling, 1995; Jamieson *et al.*, 1999). McIvor and Barry (1998a; 1998b) also found desistance came with motivation to stop, a desire to avoid incarceration, the impact on one's family, positive relationships, employment and education opportunities and a feeling of getting older. Whilst none of the desisters mentioned 'growing up' as a specific reason for stopping offending, this justification received prominence in many of the sample's reasons why *other* young people stopped offending in their early twenties. These responses support the desistance literature (Rutherford, 1986; Gottfredson and Hirschi, 1990; Moffitt, 1993) which suggests that the most common explanation for desistance is that young people 'grow out of' crime or 'grow up'. Realization was a factor closely associated with growing up and was often mentioned concurrently as to why young people stopped offending, namely, that they became more aware of the pitfalls of offending or wanted to be more conventional or 'settle down' as they got older:

> I really think that's when people are peaking, growing up, getting to the adult stage ... [You stop] because of things in your life. Different things make them realize they can't carry on like that.
>
> (Cathy, 23)

> ... you're just starting to realize, you know, maybe it's not all worth it. It's time to settle down. Staying off alcohol, staying off drugs, finding the right person.
>
> (John, 23)

> I think they just get old enough to realize it's just a nuisance. I've got a huge record and my life doesn't feel as though it's mine anymore because I'm facing the threat of the police on my back, somebody looking for you, somebody in a wig deciding what's right for you and what's not right for you.
>
> (Martin, 24)

Nevertheless, their explanations regarding 'growing up' suggest maturation and adulthood rather than age *per se*. Whilst the effect of the 'hassle factor' connected with offending was strong for many respondents, the key motivating force for desisting – or wanting to desist – came from the practical, cognitive factors of realization and reassessment. Twenty-eight of the sample of 40 implied that both they themselves and other young people who stop offending were indeed getting older or 'growing up', suggesting that offending is a 'childhood' or youthful activity:

> I've grown up ... My attitude's totally changed. I mean, I've grown up a lot since I came in here [prison]. Before I was like, em, mentally immature ... If I had a problem with anybody or an argument, I would solve it with my fist because I could handle

myself ... that's not the way to do it like. That just doesn't solve anything. That makes matters worse.

(Nick, 28)

However, rarely was this ageing process seen as the only factor influencing desistance. There was always an additional catalyst, whether this be a change of attitude or a change of circumstance.

Conclusions

This chapter has explored young people's perceptions of why they stop offending, what factors influence them and what the implications are for them of making that decision to desist from crime. In childhood and early youth, offending and the attention or influence of friends became crucial sources of capital for these young people, during a time when they possibly lacked attention, protection or encouragement from family or the wider community. Although the family can be a renewed and enduring source of support and social capital for young people as they get older (Gillies et al., 2002; Webster et al., 2004), it does nevertheless seem the case that in the youth phase, the friendship group takes precedence over the family as a means of consolidating and reinforcing one's own identity within a social setting. In later youth and early adulthood, on the other hand, the criminal justice system tended to erode what little capital accumulation they had gained from offending or indeed from conventional activities or relationships in the past. Nevertheless, opportunities for renewed family contact, relationships with conventional partners and employment or other forms of legitimate income and responsibility were a major source of capital accumulation for those young people who had left the confines of the criminal justice system and desisted from offending.

The data from this study suggest that there is no obvious turning point or time when an offender moves from the maintenance to the desistance stage. As many authors have suggested, it can be a cyclical or zig-zag path towards eventual desistance. However, what was interesting about these young people's perceptions of desistance was the fact that it was very much their decision to stop, albeit with the help and encouragement of significant others or changed circumstances. The need for friends, attention and an identity in their younger lives had encouraged them to experiment with offending. The increasing success of offending, in terms of gaining social, economic, cultural and symbolic capital, had encouraged them to continue offending for several years through adolescence and into early adulthood. For many their earlier experimentation with offending had latterly resulted in imprisonment, a distancing from family and friends and stigmatization in their communities. It was the losses and the stigma attached to offending, the growing realization of the adverse effects that offending might have on their futures, and the support and opportunities offered by significant others in their lives which eventually gave many of these young people the impetus to desist from offending.

Capital accumulation of a different or 'conventional' kind (through employment or renewing family relationships, for example) tended also to result in a reduction of offending behaviour in adulthood for several reasons. Capital could be gained from conventional or legitimate sources through opportunities to take on responsibilities, or to break with past associates, thus making offending less attractive. There tended to be a renewed emphasis on the need for family support and a greater empathy with one's parent(s). Meeting a non-offending partner was also a social catalyst to a reduction or cessation of offending behaviour.

The two key factors associated with desistance for these young people tended to be practical or relational: that is, criminal justice system 'fatigue' or because of relationships with, or the support of, family, friends and significant others. Whilst many of these factors support the theoretical evidence on desistance, there are certain anomalies. For example, the majority of the sample managed to stop offending even though they were neither in a stable relationship nor in employment. Many reasons given for stopping offending were reactive or resulting from adverse experiences rather than proactive or resulting from encouragement or practical opportunities. The majority of these respondents suggested that they made an active decision to stop offending because of the loss of control in their lives resulting from the restrictions placed on them by their reputation and lifestyle. Whilst they may have drifted *into* offending in childhood, their agency and determination to leave such a lifestyle in early adulthood was particularly strong, given that this decision meant giving up something that they were accustomed to, successful in or addicted to. There were few, if any, 'pull' factors involved, and this made their resolve all the more powerful. The fact that the majority of these young people had indeed stopped offending despite this lack of positive incentives for desistance to occur – and more importantly, to be sustained – is an anomaly which is discussed in greater depth in the following chapter. Chapter 7 draws together the common factors between youth transitions and the three phases of onset, maintenance and desistance and argues that not only can these common threads help to explain the different stages through which young people go as they move towards adulthood but they can also go some way towards identifying the factors which influence young people's propensity or otherwise to offend during this process of transition.

Chapter 7

In search of social recognition

I'd love to be able to go back until I was like about seven – six or seven ... I wouldn't take drugs at such an early age. I wouldn't offend. I'd try and be myself with people ... instead of being somebody different ... I was playing a role that I thought would fit in, but it didn't.

(Pete, 19)

Introduction

Underlying the last three chapters have been Bourdieu's concepts of capital, habitus, field and strategy, and these concepts have been used to illustrate the ways in which offending behaviour can be seen as part of one's social practice that offers various forms of capital accumulation in the transition to adulthood. The phases of transition could be seen as fields within which children and young people live out, test and modify their habitus through their social practice and it is suggested that offending is one strategy which young people with limited capital may adopt to gain greater recognition in that transition. Young people place increasing value on friends and family in the process of growing up. Their culture and social world are but a microcosm within the wider society, but Bourdieu's notion of capital offers a common denominator between the microcosmic world of young people in transition and the macrocosmic world of 'mainstream' society.

Bourdieu's concepts of capital are crucial in linking the phases of transition with the three phases identified in offending histories – onset, maintenance and desistance. The period of youth is one where boundaries are blurred, guidance and support are often reduced or passing from one source (the family) to another (the friendship group), and responsibilities are not wholly acknowledged as legitimate or sustainable. This phase in the transition is the one in which most offending takes place. Youth is the phase when young people have few socially recognized means of legitimating their stake in the social world but may see offending or its benefits as their only means of gaining recognition meantime, even if such recognition comes only from their friends. However, what is missing from this analysis is the answer to the question of how capital in its various forms can reduce the likelihood of offending when such capital can be gained from offending itself. The answer, I believe, may lie in the concept of 'social recognition', where a combination of *expenditure* and accumulation of capital is necessary not only in the transition to adulthood but also in the transition to desistance. This adaptation and development of Bourdieu's concepts of capital is explored further in this penultimate chapter.

The case studies drawn on in the previous three chapters illustrate the experiences and perceptions of the majority of the young people in this research. What emerges from these accounts is the seeming lack of continuity or stability in these young people's lives and their desire throughout childhood and into adulthood for interaction and integration within society, whether this be through family, friends, partners or employment. Pete, Laura, Anna and Yvonne, for example, spoke of the trauma in childhood of moving from somewhere familiar into a new or strange environment, because of a change of home area or school. These moves tended to coincide with a feeling of isolation or instability, resulting in the need to counteract this with the making of new friends, however disruptive those friendships may have been. Pete, Vic, Laura and Yvonne spoke of bereavement, familial abuse or separation from one or both parents, and many others in the study spoke of the lack of care or attention they received from their parents in childhood. All of these factors demonstrated a lack of capital for these young people and such factors were often suggested to be major influences in their propensity to offend.

It was suggested in Chapter 3 that the three phases of transition (childhood, youth and adulthood) could be seen as 'fields' according to Bourdieu's definition of field. They are sites of struggle between competing forces of power, both within and between each phase of transition. In childhood, for example, offending could be seen as a means of gaining power within the friendship group when other sources of capital are either dissipating (through a distancing from the family unit) or changing (through the entrance into an adult-led and authoritarian school environment or through the development of an individual and social identity). Either way, children from disadvantaged backgrounds or those lacking confidence or emotional support, may well feel vulnerable in such changed circumstances. In youth, if offending proves successful in accumulating more, or sustaining existing capital, such behaviour is likely to be continued, not least if alternative sources of capital are elusive, denied or rejected. Only when offending is seen to have more social costs than personal benefits will young people attempt to modify their behaviour so as to adapt to their current social situation.

A lack of capital in one's life tends to manifest itself as a pervasive undercurrent, rather than being triggered by specific circumstances. Thus, there is not always a 'trigger event' that propels these young people into or out of offending. Some eventually leave it for proactive reasons (having gained capital from legitimate sources, for example). Others leave it for reactive reasons, for example because the symbolic capital denied them, as a result of involvement in the criminal justice system or their wider reputation as offenders, outweighs the actual benefits of offending. Once young people reach the age of 16, and assuming they are detected in their offending, the criminal justice system may then interrupt the flow of social, economic, cultural and symbolic capital they can accrue. Over time, their involvement with the criminal justice system may erode what little capital they have already accumulated, even though such involvement may have initially enhanced their access to social and symbolic capital within their friendship groups.

The vast majority of respondents mentioned friendships as being important to them at this time of personal change and social development, and the majority talked of offending as a means towards gaining or sustaining such friendships. However, for the women, it would seem that the need for identity within the social group extended beyond the phase of onset into the phase of maintenance of offending through the influence of boyfriends, as illustrated by both Laura and Anna in particular. It was through these relationships, often with men much older than themselves, that many of the women gained attention and love, even though a mutual drug habit was often the catalyst to their sustaining, or persevering in, such relationships. Gilligan (1982) argues that in adolescence, young women confuse identity and intimacy and define their own identity through their relationships with others, whether or not this be through the medium of drugs. The men, on the other hand, seemed to be less rather than more dependent on friends or partners as they got older, and relied more on the economic and symbolic capital that money and reputation gave them.

Several respondents found renewed sanctuary within family relationships at the time of stopping or attempting to stop offending, relationships that had often hitherto been problematic (for example, Laura, Pete and Anna). It has been argued (Gillies *et al.*, 2002; Jones and Wallace, 1992; Thomson *et al.*, 2003) that there is a lack of importance given to family and other relationships in theories of individualization in late modernity, given that much recent research on young people's narratives has stressed the influence of family in the transition to adulthood:

> While young people constructed adult status in terms of independence and personal responsibility, the enduring significance of relationships with parents was also emphasized ... the majority of young people in our sample still valued and relied on a close relationship with their parents. The knowledge that parents are available to provide emotional and practical support when needed appeared to be particularly appreciated.
> (Gillies *et al.*, 2002: 43)

For many of the young people with an addiction, giving up drugs or alcohol, like stopping offending, required the support and encouragement of others (in terms of social or symbolic capital in particular), as evidenced by Laura, Pete and Yvonne. Equally, methadone was an important source of capital during the process of stopping offending in that it relieved the symptoms of withdrawal, was free on prescription and enabled greater stability and continuity within their lives. It would seem from these accounts that the need for increased capital of whatever form was important to both the men and the women in childhood but that as they progressed through the youth phase and into adulthood there was a gendered divergence: the women were more likely to value increased or sustained social capital in particular, whilst the men were more likely to value increased or sustained symbolic capital. This finding supports the contention by Chodorow (Gilligan, 1982: 7) that 'feminine personality comes to define itself in relation and connection to other people more than masculine personality does'. However, it was not possible in the current research to explore the extent to which societal expectations of gendered roles influenced these young people's propensity to accumulate one or other form of capital.

As is the contention throughout this book, young people may use offending as a means of gaining recognition, attention, income or friends, not least at a time when other sources of capital accumulation are beyond their reach or in limited supply. For those who stopped offending in their twenties, many had found opportunities to accumulate capital through means other than offending, opportunities which did not result in criminal justice system involvement, a lack of control or wider social disapproval. Such opportunities for capital accumulation included improved family relationships, not being dependent on illegal drugs, having a job or their own tenancy and being a parent themselves. However, it is acknowledged that many who had *not* stopped offending also had access to such opportunities for accumulating capital but were unable or unwilling, for varying reasons, to desist from crime. This anomaly has been a major source of concern for criminologists, as was seen in Chapter 2, and suggests that capital accumulation on its own cannot account for desistance. This chapter further develops the concept of capital in order to provide a possible solution to this anomaly.

It is therefore suggested in this chapter that capital expenditure[1] is a missing link in the chain of events surrounding both youth transitions and youth offending and that 'social recognition' – namely, the attainment of a combination of accumulation and expenditure of social, economic, cultural and symbolic capital that is both durable and legitimated – is a possible way forward in understanding the temporary nature of much youth crime. Whilst capital accumulation is a crucial factor in aiding both desistance *and* a smoother transition to adulthood, the added factor of capital expenditure is required to ensure that young people have not only the opportunity and incentive to desist from crime but also the longer-term opportunities afforded their counterparts in adulthood. Social recognition can be a helpful concept in understanding desistance amongst young people in transition because it expresses the capacity and need that young people have for longer-term *reciprocal* relations of trust and responsibility within the wider society.

Expenditure versus accumulation of capital

Bourdieu (1997; 1998) has argued that only in durable circumstances will capital accumulate and reproduce itself. However, in youth transitions, such durable circumstances are, by definition, unlikely given the transient and 'liminal' status of young people in the youth phase. Skeggs (1997) argues that capital can only be 'capitalized' upon if it is convertible ('traded up') in an institutionalized setting through lawful authority (ibid.: 161), for example, through converting cultural capital (qualifications) into economic capital (better employment prospects) and symbolic capital (academic recognition). Young people generally, because of a lack of opportunities for wider societal responsibility and because of their limited legal and social status as adults, have less capital which is legitimate, convertible and, therefore, tradeable, not least for young people from working class backgrounds (Skeggs, 1997). It is acknowledged here that many young people, notably those from middle class backgrounds, have the opportunities and resources to both accumulate and spend capital. Equally, many young people as well as adults do *not* have these opportunities and resources because of structural constraints. However, without status, resources and rights in the adult world, many young people are unlikely to gain the legitimacy or convertibility of capital: what capital they accumulate tends only to be recognized in the eyes of their immediate social network rather than being given wider social recognition.

Bourdieu suggests that individuals' identities are flexible and dynamic – 'nothing classifies somebody more than the way he or she classifies' (1989, quoted in Haugaard, 2002: 237). In other words, individuals behave in ways that 'fit' with their social position. However, Bourdieu sees social positions *per se* as relatively rigid and static, and again this denies the fluid and changing situation for young people in transition. Skeggs (1997: 94) agrees with Bourdieu to the extent that 'identities are continually in the process of being re-produced as responses to social positions', but she found in her study of working class women that they did not adjust to their social positions, as Bourdieu might suggest. On the contrary, 'they made strenuous efforts to deny, disidentify and dissimulate' (ibid.: 94). This suggests that individuals have greater agency to determine their 'ideal' social position, rather than having this determined for them by structural constraints. Skeggs also argues that whilst there are differential amounts and distributions of the various forms of capital within a society, for working class women such capital has limited availability and market value.

Accumulation of capital for the young people in my study was achieved through, *inter alia*, having a reputation amongst their peers, through becoming involved in friendships or relationships, through making money from crime or employment and through having children. As they got older and took on greater responsibilities for themselves or others (e.g. through caring for partners or children or gaining employment), the opportunities for expenditure became more accessible to them. Nevertheless, such expenditure of capital was more difficult to achieve in either the childhood or youth phase, by dint of their age, liminal status and relative powerlessness.

Opportunities for capital expenditure in the desistance phase

Instances of accumulation of capital often far outweighed those of expenditure for these young people, and yet it was the expenditure of capital as they got older that gave these young people a strong sense of achievement and was more likely to encourage desistance. Table 7.1 suggests some instances where legitimate expenditure was achieved by the desisters in this study. Whilst acknowledging that some of the persisters had also had opportunities for the expenditure of capital in childhood and youth, it is suggested here that either there were no sustained opportunities for the expenditure of capital, or the outlets for such capital were not of a legitimate nature. In other words, some of the opportunities for expenditure of capital described in Table 7.1 may well have arisen in the childhood and youth phases, but these opportunities tended to be short-lived and based on the recognition or legitimation of friends and family rather than the wider society. As the young people moved into the more public arena of adulthood, however, a combination of accumulation and expenditure of capital which was both durable and legitimated was more likely to occur.

Whereas economic capital can be spent on goods and services as well as on people, the expenditure of the three other forms of capital – social, cultural and symbolic – is mainly achievable in relation to people. The focus of this chapter is on the broader *social* aspect of capital expenditure since it is argued here that such interdependence and reciprocity are crucial in achieving social recognition. In this

Table 7.1 Expenditure of capital associated with desistance

Capital	
Social	• having responsibilities to one's family, partner or children • becoming a parent • giving love, friendship or attention to others • seeking custody of one's child
Economic	• 'buying' clothes and other consumables (as opposed to stealing them) • spending money on one's house or children • paying taxes and other state contributions
Cultural	• contributing towards others' development or welfare through employment, teaching or influence, based on one's own skills or experience • setting an example by one's actions or words • encouraging and helping others
Symbolic	• wanting to give of oneself (as mentor, volunteer, worker, etc.) • wanting to offer restoration/reparation to the community • having responsibilities towards one's house or job

respect, two key models of interdependence and reciprocity, taking on responsibility and generativity, which allow for opportunities for expenditure of social, cultural and symbolic capital, are examined in the following section. This section, however, concludes with a brief summary of the expenditure potential of economic capital in relation to this sample.

Having income from employment enabled some of these respondents not only to earn money but also to spend money that had not been gained by illegal means, often for the first time in their lives. For those who had given up drugs as well as offending or for those who had latterly been prescribed methadone, the very fact of not having to spend their money on drugs, but being able instead to spend such money on household items, was often seen as a novelty. In short, they spoke of their pride at being able not only to accumulate, but also to spend 'honest' money on 'normal' things:

> I've bought things that are in my wardrobe. I've bought all my Christmas presents. That makes me feel good.
>
> (Nina, 23)

> I can hold my head up high. I'm not ashamed of myself. I've got more self-worth now ... I've worked a week for my money, my money's mine to spend, the stuff I buy [my son] isn't stuff that I've stolen ... He never wanted for anything, but ... I feel better now buying him something ...
>
> (Gillian, 29)

The main function of economic capital for young people seems to be as a means of gaining increased symbolic capital (through being able to buy 'designer' or other desirable consumer goods) rather than as a financial investment for the future. As such, young people with seemingly few prospects for spending capital in reciprocal ways may resort to conspicuous consumption rather than deferred gratification. As Fukuyama (1995) has pointed out in relation to the importance of employment for gaining capital:

> Our motivation in working and earning money is much more closely related to the recognition that such activity affords us, where money becomes a symbol not for material goods but for social status or recognition.
>
> (Fukuyama, 1995: 359)

Many respondents mentioned first-hand experience of poverty as children and some suggested that being placed in the care of the local authority was a relatively more secure means of ensuring access to economic capital than the family home (through clothing allowances, increased pocket money, etc.). But again, this economic gain was symbolic in that it gave them access to status rather than financial power *per se*. Many of the respondents also suggested that the need or desire for money as children was an incentive to starting offending, and some calculated that the financial benefits of offending often far outweighed the costs.

Although the expenditure capacity of economic capital is crucial in the transition to adulthood, it has limited potential for young people who are unlikely to gain sustained employment in early adulthood, when desistance is likely to occur. It is thus to the other three forms of capital that this chapter now turns. The two main forms of expenditure with regard to social, cultural and symbolic capital are 'taking on responsibility' and 'generativity'. These are described briefly below before interweaving the views of the young people in this analysis.

Taking on responsibility

There are subtle nuances in the meaning of the word 'responsibility'. It can mean 'having responsibility' which suggests being accountable (to someone) for something; 'acting responsibly' where expectations are placed on the actor by others; or alternatively 'taking on responsibility' which suggests the opportunity of being trusted with something for someone. Farrall and Bowling (1997: 22) describe responsibility as:

> an identity which entails behaving in a particular manner. This manner represents the duality of structure, in that the social identity of 'responsibility' is both prior to the individual and dependent upon individual actions and decisions.

These authors equate responsibility with Giddens' (1984) notion of both 'rules' (legal or social expectations) and 'resources' (a desire for accountability or caring for others). Qualitative studies of young people have implied that both rules and resources influence their feelings of responsibility (Barry, 2001a, 2001b; Dearden and Becker, 2000; Farrall and Bowling, 1997; Graham and Bowling, 1995; Holland *et al.*, 1999), and this study is no exception, as the quotations cited below illustrate. Whilst the young people took on responsibility as both an expectation and a desire, in this section I particularly want to stress the 'resource' implications of taking on responsibility, namely, having the desire, the opportunity, the capacity and the incentive to be trusted with a task of benefit to significant others. Many adults – as well as some young people themselves (Barry, 2001a) – may see responsibility taking by children in particular as a burden inappropriate to their age and status. However, others see such responsibility taking as emancipatory and participatory, although the level and intensity of such responsibility need to be tempered with the capacities and wishes of the child (Franklin, 2002; Archard, 1993).

It has been suggested by several authors that young people tend not to equate adulthood with rights *per se* but with personal responsibility (Barry, 2001b; Gillies *et al.*, 2002; Lister *et al.*, 2002). A study by Holland *et al.* (1999) suggests that young people view responsibility as one of the defining positive features of adulthood, not least in relation to a sense of responsibility towards their families. Based on their sample of adolescents, Holland *et al.* suggest that feelings of obligation towards parents and other family members become more prominent as young people become older. Equally, Dearden and Becker (2000) in their study of young carers, suggest that young people consider responsibility as a positive asset in terms of caring for others and learning new skills. Farrall and Bowling (1997), in an analysis of the interplay between agency and structure in young people's propensity or otherwise to stop offending, imply that taking on responsibility for one's family or oneself has a positive impact on the likelihood of desistance. These authors suggest that social identities in adulthood incorporate both rights and responsibilities, and that such identities require the fulfilment of certain roles, the adherence to certain rules (responsibility is not compatible with offending behaviour) and the management of resources (achieving adult goals).

Employment was seen as a crucial arena in which the young people in this sample could gain social status through taking on responsibility, with 17 young men and 14 young women mentioning their desire for a job in the future. This is not an unusual finding, given the emphasis placed on employment by young people generally in the transition to adulthood as a means of gaining status, rights and stability (see, for example, Barry, 2001b; Stephen, 2000).

For the majority of this sample, their main responsibility was to their current partners (9 men and 7 women) or to their children (6 men and 15 women). Equal emphasis was placed by both male and female respondents on responsibilities towards people (including themselves) as well as towards practicalities, such as a tenancy, paying bills, a job and to remain offence- or drug-free in the future:

> I've got a responsibility to myself, to keep myself out of trouble and off drugs and I've got my baby on its way. I've got a responsibility towards [my partner] as well ... Attend probation, hospital, lawyers.
>
> (Sarah, 27)

> Just making [my fiancé] happy. I love that. I get all excited when he comes home. I like doing his cooking but I wish I had more responsibility. I've got responsibilities to try and be a mum again. That's a responsibility. [MB: *What other responsibilities would you like?*] A job. Getting up every morning. Working for a living.
>
> (Yvonne, 25)

I decided that it was time to wake up and realize what I've got and what I would lose. I've got my wee laddie and that ... I had enough of going around and getting lifted by the police and that ... if I go down, I'm going to lose the life of my son growing up and things like that ... I had my girlfriend, I had my son, my family.

(Frank, 22)

One young man went as far as to say he also had responsibilities towards the wider society, epitomizing Giddens' definition (1984: 18) of responsibility as a 'rule' or legal or moral expectation within society:

Responsibility to the public and, you know, society as a whole. I mean, I can't go round thumping society ... I can't go round using my fists all the time. I can't keep committing crime. I can't do it. Society won't stand for it.

(Nick, 28)

Finally, four men out of the total sample of 40 young people considered that they had no current responsibilities – three were in prison at the time of the interview and the remaining one was living with his parents[2]:

I did have responsibility for a house and a job, but I've no responsibilities now.

(Kevin, 23, interviewed in prison)

I've nothing. No house, no kids, nothing.

(Len, 26, interviewed in prison)

Generativity

Erikson (1968: 141) coined the phrase 'generativity' to mean a passing on of care, attention and support to future generations based on one's own experiences. McAdams and de St Aubin (1998) describe the term as: 'The concern for and commitment to promoting the next generation, manifested through parenting, teaching, mentoring ... ' (quoted in Maruna, 2001: 99). Generativity suggests the expenditure of cultural and social capital in particular. However, these young people had little access to institutionalized cultural capital (Skeggs,

1997), in the sense of educational attainment, qualifications or legitimate competence, not least because of their young age, their seeming disaffection from the educational system and their lack of rights and responsibilities as adults. The few qualifications they did have were often deemed by them to have been undermined by their criminal records and reputation, and therefore seemed of little use to them in the future. Equally, the skills and competences gained in childhood and youth – their sources of cultural capital – are often not recognized or legitimated by adults and tend, therefore, to go undetected (Barry, 2001b). As Bromley points out:

> Failure to establish an approved role in society, through educational failure and unemployment for example, leads some people to suppose that they have little to lose from antisocial behaviour. This applies especially if their social network consists of people of a similar kind. Consequently, threats to their wider reputation through misconduct may have little or no effect on behaviour. Conversely, people with an established approved role in society have a lot to lose.
>
> (Bromley, 1993: 62)

Five of the men and three of the women in this study specifically stated that they were interested in the caring professions (social work or counselling, for example) as a result of their own skills and experiences in the past. A further two already had experience of employment as drugs counsellors. Their wish to give of their own skills or experience to benefit others illustrates a feeling of generativity:

> I'd love to be a drugs counsellor, I would. I really would. I'd love to be able to sit with a group of people and talk to them. It is, it's a shame. I've been through it all myself.
>
> (Anna, 21)

> I want to be an instructor for an outward bound course. I want to put into the community what I've taken from it. I want to do courses with under-privileged kids like myself.
>
> (Nick, 28)

> ... maybe get a really good job in the social work or something like that ... I get on with the younger ones up here and I try and

say to them – don't do what I done, stop taking that [drugs] because it ruins everything.

(Bernadette, 23)

Sixteen of the women and seven of the men mentioned at interview that they had children. McRobbie (2000: 206) suggests that young women, notably those with no immediate employment prospects or other sources of capital accumulation, may choose motherhood as a positive option:

For girls who had never been brought up to consider themselves as wage-earners, never mind career women, bringing forward motherhood by a few years was hardly a surprising step, indeed it was from their point of view a resourceful activity.

Craine (1997) acknowledges that motherhood may bring social and housing stability in the short term, thus easing at least one aspect of the transition to adulthood. Nevertheless, he argues that: 'early domestic careers of pregnancy, childrearing and home-caring served, typically, to locate young women in situations of economic and often domestic, subordination' (ibid.: 143). In addition, as highlighted by recent cultural criminological research, the attraction of motherhood as an alternative occupation for young women with few other legitimate opportunities in the transition to adulthood, has been vilified in the media as rejecting family values, being sexually promiscuous and misusing welfare benefits (McRobbie, 2000; Rolfe, 2005).

Many respondents saw parenthood as a positive choice for them, and several commented that they wished to be better parents than their own parents had been, to ensure that their own children were not compromised as they had been. Interestingly, the fathers in the study voiced greater concerns in this respect than the mothers:

My main goal is to watch my kids grow up healthy and keep them away from drugs.

(Harry, 26)

I'm teaching my kids to be nothing like this. My kids won't be like that.

(Vic, 23)

> Making sure that [my daughter] gets the things that I never got in life, like a good home, steady family, mother and father to care for her, good schooling, you know. Just make opportunities for her.
>
> (Nick, 28)

One of the mothers feared for the safety of her own daughter, having been abused herself at a young age. Her need to protect her child illustrates a generative expenditure of social and cultural capital:

> 'cos she's a girl as well and I feel as if I've got to be there 24 hours a day to protect her but I know if she's with [my partner], I know she's alright when she's with him.
>
> (Diane, 21)

Maruna (2001) stresses the importance of generativity not only in being constructive for others but also in being cathartic and purposeful for oneself in helping break a cycle of offending. He identifies four reasons for this:

- fulfilment (giving the individual meaning and a sense of achievement);
- restitution (giving the individual relief from a sense of shame or guilt);
- legitimacy (giving the individual social credibility); and
- therapy (reinforcing the individual's determination to reform).

Whilst Maruna's study of current and ex-offenders illustrated examples of all four reasons for generativity, the present sample tended to emphasize only two – fulfilment and legitimacy. As far as therapy and restitution are concerned, few of the young people mentioned a sense of reflection, guilt or shame in relation to feelings of generativity. When talking about offering their own experience and knowledge to help others in similar circumstances to themselves, it was more because of a belief that such experience and knowledge were still valuable tools in retrospect. They took a more pragmatic rather than 'restitutive' approach which focused more on preventive measures for other young people than on rehabilitative measures for themselves. However, this line of reasoning is tentative since it was not explored at interview. Nevertheless, it would merit further research, not least given the wide range of literature which supports a shaming, reformative or therapeutic angle to changing one's behaviour or lifestyle (see Maruna, 2001 for a résumé of such literature).

If young people have greater opportunities to take on responsibilities, they can accumulate social, cultural and symbolic capital through being needed, trusted and respected. In addition, they can also spend such capital through taking on a caring or responsible role and giving of themselves to generative activities as a means of paying back the community for past offending (see, for example, Braithwaite, 1989). Maruna (2001) found the influence of generativity emerging in the career aspirations of the current and ex-offenders within his sample who were keen to help others in similar situations to themselves.[3] McIvor (1992) also commented on the therapeutic effects of community service on offenders, notably when they were actively helping others and could see the direct benefits of their work to recipients.

In summary, taking on responsibilities and generativity are crucial factors in the development and sustainability of social recognition. Responsibility towards other people (e.g. through a caring or loving relationship) or towards oneself (e.g. in maintaining a tenancy or holding down a job) gives young people the legitimacy and opportunity to spend as well as accumulate capital within the wider society. Equally, generativity offers both fulfilment, interdependence and legitimacy, the latter of which in particular is an essential element of ensuring ultimate social recognition.

Examples of expenditure of capital

The following six case study summaries – the three persisters and three desisters cited in Chapters 4, 5 and 6 – exemplify the levels of capital expenditure available to many of the young people in the research. This analysis is secondary and the issue of expenditure of capital was not specifically addressed at interview, although respondents were asked questions regarding the responsibilities they currently had and what they would lose if they were to continue offending in the future. The following summary tables briefly explore the types of capital these young people were spending through taking on responsibility or through generativity.

Yvonne, 25, desister

Social	Seeking custody of her daughter; having responsibilities to her fiancé
Economic	None identified
Cultural	Caring for her terminally ill mother
Symbolic	Responsibilities to her house; (potential) responsibilities to a job

Yvonne stopped offending when she met her fiancé, and implied that the act of stopping offending was one that required expenditure of capital: *'You can see you're hurting someone else ... I had to [stop offending] if I wanted to keep [my fiancé]. He wouldnae have stayed around ... I don't want to lose him. He means too much. He's done too much.'* Likewise, she had to stop offending in order to prove that she could be a mother again to her daughter: *'I miss seeing her; I've not really seen her for a year ... It's making me realize what an idiot I've been. I've missed out on a lot. I think she's gonna be my strongest part ... I've got responsibilities to try and be a mum again. That's a responsibility'.* Although Yvonne did not have a job at the time of interview, she hoped to find one after her wedding that year, since this would give her the increased responsibility that she wanted in her changed life: *'A job. Getting up every morning. Working for a living.'* Meantime, she was spending cultural and emotional capital caring for her mother who had cancer. She decided to renew her relationship with her mother – one that had been, she thought, non-existent in her childhood – when she heard that her mother was terminally ill and needed her support. Although there was still friction between the two of them, and she felt this was damaging her relationship with her fiancé, Yvonne nevertheless continued to visit her mother and support her in whatever ways she could: *'She's been through a lot, she's had all these big operations, but she's still drinking and smoking ... [and] hurting me. She doesn't really give a damn about anybody or anything.'* Her main responsibilities, however, were to her daughter, and the pending court case for custody, and to her fiancé: *'Just making [him] happy. I love that. I get all excited when he comes home. I like doing his cooking.'*

Pete, 19, desister

Social	Responsibilities to his current girlfriend and his family
Economic	Paying off debts
Cultural	Concern for his (ex-)girlfriends
Symbolic	Responsibilities to his house

Pete's main responsibilities currently were to his house (he had his own tenancy), to his pet dog, to his girlfriend and to his family – in that order! Previous bereavements (two girlfriends had miscarriages) and latterly splitting up with these two girlfriends had given him a greater awareness of and concern for other people's needs: *'The loss of my kids made me think a lot more. And the loss of two people I loved, my girlfriends. I've got feelings for my girlfriends. That made me think an awful lot, like.'* His mother had been a strong source of support for Pete when he overcame a heroin addiction recently (thus spending her own cultural and social capital on her son) and he felt a need to repay that support when necessary: *'Just to be there if I'm needed.'*

At the end of the interview, Pete offered further advice for professionals working with young people which demonstrates the need for expenditure of capital. He spoke at length about how young people generally could be helped to stop offending, and implied that opportunities to prove themselves through taking on responsibility were an important factor: *'Give young people ... give them somewhere they can go and do something. Open up more chances for them getting jobs after school and stuff like that, you know. Give them community stuff they can do like get all the kids in the community to build a park like in the town. Build a skateboard run ... Give them something that's gonna help the community'.* He also implied that the expenditure of cultural capital by professionals (e.g. the caring nature of social work) required first-hand knowledge of the problems faced by young people: *'[Get] folk who understand what they're going through to talk to them ... Having somebody there that's done it. That's what's wrong with care, a lot of the people that are care workers and that are all folk who've been brought up in a good home, they've been to a good school, they've had everything paid for until they're 16, and they've gone out and got work straightaway and that, and they've got their life sorted. They don't understand what it's like to be unemployed, to be on the dole, to be in jail or care or anywhere like that, you know. And folk who understand it can sit there and say to the kids "now look, I've been there, I've done exactly what you're doing and this is the way it will end up". You know what I mean? They need more experience in the care system about offending and stuff like that.'*

Laura, 27, desister

Social	Responsibilities to her two children and her family
Economic	Responsibilities to pay the bills
Cultural	Concern not to hurt her children further
Symbolic	Responsibilities to her house

Laura spoke of her pride at having both her children, and how important they were to her now, since she nearly died from an overdose two years prior to interview. It was her responsibilities to her children that made her decide to stop offending: *'I near died and like, you know, support machine and everything ... so it gave me a fright ... The thought of ... my kids not seeing me again ... So the thought of that, you know what I mean, actually freaked me out.'* Now on a methadone prescription, Laura was working towards reducing the dosage and her aspirations for the future were to *'see my kids settled and happy'*, through the expenditure of her own cultural, social and symbolic capital. Although she did not have employment, the fact that she had given up illicit drugs meant that she could spend economic capital (from benefits) looking after her house and children, rather than on drugs.

Vic, 23, persister

Social   Responsibilities to his mother
Economic   None identified
Cultural   (Potential) concern for the upbringing of his
            children
Symbolic   None identified

Vic was in prison at the time of the interview, and seemed resigned to further periods of incarceration. When asked whether he had any responsibilities currently, his first reaction was '*none*', but he then suggested that he had responsibilities to his mother: '*just to keep my nose clean*', even though he implied that his mother was as resigned to his continued offending as he was himself. Vic suggested, hypothetically, that if he found a job, settled down and had a child, it might help him to stop offending, but he could not readily suggest ways in which he could or would give to others (in terms of capital expenditure), other than the comment that if he had children in the future: '*I'm teaching my kids to be nothing like this.*' The fact that he had spent the major part of his youth in prison suggested that Vic had had little opportunity to make or sustain close social networks through which to spend capital. His success (in terms of immediate monetary gains) from offending also made the prospect of legitimate employment less attractive to him.

Anna, 21, persister

Social   Seeking custody of her daughter
Economic   None identified
Cultural   Desire to become a drugs counsellor
Symbolic   None identified

Anna's offending was influenced by both alcohol and friends who were offending; she also had court cases pending as well as the custody battle for her daughter, both of which made planning for the future more difficult in terms of capital expenditure. She had been told by the social work department that she would not get her daughter back for at least five years. Meantime, her only responsibility was to stay off drugs, so as to prove to the social work department that she would be capable of caring for her daughter in five years' time: a tall order perhaps for someone with little other incentive to keep going. Anna wanted to move area if and when she got her daughter back, partly to sever all ties with her ex-boyfriend, but meantime she had to live locally to where her daughter was placed in care. Anna suggested that getting her daughter back eventually would be a positive incentive to stopping offending and coming off drugs. In terms of generativity through employment, Anna said that she wanted to become a drugs counsellor in the future, given her own experience of drug addiction in the past.

Derek, 21, persister

Social	Responsibility towards his parents and siblings
Economic	Investing in a new relationship
Cultural	None identified
Symbolic	None identified

Derek came from a close family background and felt increasing responsibility, as the oldest child, towards his parents and younger sisters as he got older. Although Derek was working part-time for his father, it was casual labour and he would have preferred stable employment: *'Earning a wage feels brilliant, man'*. However, he suggested that his criminal record was a liability in this respect.

Derek said he needed to control his temper and strengthen his resolve not to *'play the hard man'* in order to be able to stop offending: *'I'm slowly but surely getting there, ken ... I'm sick of it ... I'll get my own flat.'* However, the external constraints to capital expenditure were pending court cases, the likelihood of a prison sentence and the lack of full-time employment. He suggested that he could not find employment or his own tenancy until he had '*a clean slate*'. He was also, at the time of interview, trying to consolidate a relationship with a new girlfriend and to impress her, thereby spending capital on her, but felt restrained by his lack of income: '*I'm trying to get together with a girl now. She's at university and all that and I meet her, ken, and try to put the talk on and that, eh ... [Last] Saturday, man, I spent about a hundred quid on the two of us up the town – "no I'll get it, no I'll get it", ken. So if I've not got the money ... she's got money but I just don't like girls doing it [paying] unless we've been going for a while ... She'd better not just be after my money or I'll crack up.*'

Constraints to capital expenditure

Bourdieu has been criticized for being overly deterministic in suggesting that the habitus, rather than one's capital, defines and delimits one's ability to progress to new challenges and opportunities (Jenkins, 1992, although see Fowler, 2000). Whilst the conditions of existence may well be homogeneous, it has been argued by Bourdieu's critics that individuals have the agency to move beyond or to manipulate those objective conditions (MacRae, 2002; Raffo and Reeves, 2000). Nevertheless, Bourdieu argues that the field one operates within determines the boundaries of the habitus and that when fields are not well-defined entities and two or more fields overlap, a problematic blurring of boundaries is likely to occur:

> The relation between habitus and field operates in two ways. On one side, it is a relation of *conditioning*: the field structures the habitus, which is the product of the embodiment of the immanent necessity of a field (or of a set of intersecting fields, the extent of their intersection or discrepancy being at the root of a divided or even torn habitus). On the other side, it is a relation of knowledge of *cognitive construction*.
>
> (Bourdieu and Wacquant, 1992: 127, emphases in original)

These areas of overlap fit with Bourdieu's term 'intersection or discrepancy' as described in the above quotation. The extent of this overlap between fields results, as this quotation suggests, in a 'divided or even torn habitus', making movements from one habitus to another more difficult to achieve: hence, Bourdieu's contention that such movement may result in failure. Raffo and Reeves (2000) have suggested that young people can, however, have differing but overlapping individualized social networks that are often fluid and changing. They suggest that the notion of habitus can accommodate dynamic and heterogeneous social interactions, and allow for a smoother transition between and within time and place:

> ... individualized constellations of social relations are evolving and unique because the changing individual biography of a given individual, at any given time, requires different types of interaction with particular types of individuals.
>
> (Raffo and Reeves, 2000: 152)

Just as Bourdieu sees class relations as fields in their own right, age relations could equally be seen as fields, namely the fields of childhood, youth and adulthood. Thus, the claim of likely failure in the transition from one field or habitus to another holds some truth when considered in the light of the findings from this research, where young people are moving from the habitus they had developed in the field of childhood, through to the habitus they aspired to in the field of adulthood, via the habitus experienced in the field of youth. The legal and economic constraints imposed on young people by dint of their social status were difficult to overcome in early adulthood without the opportunities for reciprocal relations and responsibilities within the wider society.

As depicted in Figure 7.1, the factors that prevented these young people from spending capital could be grouped into six key areas: having liminal status in transition, being dependent on drugs, having a reputation as an offender, not having a house of one's own, being unemployed and being involved in the criminal justice system.

The lack of capital for these respondents was apparent not only from their *liminal status* as 'young people', but also because of being marginalized within the labour market and having limited rights as full citizens (Coles, 1995; Jones, 1996). The constraints to them achieving status as 'adults' included the lack of access to either income from employment or state benefits and their limited opportunities for taking on responsibility in the transition period. Whilst they may have had expectations and aspirations which mirrored mainstream norms, these were often denied them

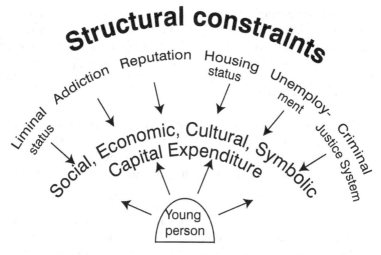

Figure 7.1 Constraints on capital expenditure

because of their status as young people. Those who were denied responsibilities towards their children because of those children being looked after elsewhere were also vulnerable to 'liminality'. Both Yvonne and Anna, for example, suggested that if they lost their battle to gain custody of their children, they were more likely to re-offend, whereas they both strongly felt that renewing their caring role with their children would have a profound influence on their ability and motivation to stop offending. These sentiments are reminiscent of Leibrich's (1993) suggestion, quoted in Chapter 2, that those with nothing to live for in effect have nothing to lose.

In the case of *drug addiction*, many respondents suggested that their drug use was problematic and constrained the development of their social and individual identities. Coming off drugs required heightened self-determination since many suggested that outside agency help was not forthcoming at the time they needed it. Equally, Vic, for example, spoke of the difficulty of stopping heroin when he could access it both in prison and in the community. However, for those who were put on methadone, they were eased away from the financial burden of obtaining illicit drugs and therefore no longer needed to offend to 'feed' a habit.

Having a *reputation* as an offender or a drug user equally exacerbated these young people's capacity to accumulate and spend capital. They spoke either of not being trusted or not being able (through, for example, ill-health resulting from an addiction) to take on responsibility, or of being unable to overcome discriminatory attitudes and practices of potential employers, the police or the local community more generally. For example, Laura stopped offending over three years prior to interview but still felt stigmatized within her local community:

> everyone would look down on me, they still actually do ... and names stick... even so now, I am a wee bit scared when I see a police car. Although I know I've not done nothing, I always feel, oh, they'll lift me for something that someone else has done.
>
> (Laura, 27)

Likewise, Vic felt resigned to his reputation, which only served to reduce his motivation to change: '[The police] expect me to do it 'cos they're used to what I'm like ... Everybody knows I'm a shoplifter'. Anna felt constrained by her past reputation locally as a drug addict: 'I'm trying to sort my head out and people aren't giving me the chance, you know. People just see me as a smackhead, down and out, junkie'. Bromley (1993), for example, describes 'primary' reputations as being based on first-hand knowledge of the holder of that reputation; whereas 'secondary' reputations are based on hearsay. Hence the importance of the immediate social environment in fostering and disseminating that reputation. Bromley suggests that developing and sustaining a 'good' primary reputation requires a social network within which that knowledge of the person can spread and be reinforced. Young people in transition, notably those disadvantaged by a lack of opportunities for social capital, are unlikely to have the social networks that can confirm their changed or developing reputations. And for those like Derek who come from neighbourhoods which expect one to offend or to be 'a hard man', it is doubly difficult to break away from the expectations of others.

Living at home was a financial necessity for some respondents, and several had returned to the family home because of an inability to cope on their own. Jones (1995) suggests that the number of young people returning home following a period of independent living had increased dramtically towards the end of the twentieth century, and that young women were more susceptible to such cyclical transitions. Whilst young people generally want to assert their individual identities by becoming independent of the parental home (Jones, 1995), working class young people in particular often do not have the financial means to sustain an independent lifestyle away from the economic support of their families. Equally, several respondents felt constrained by the area in which they were living, either because of the adverse influence of local people, because they needed to remain near to their children or because of the lack of opportunities in their local community. For example, Derek suggested that he would have to move area to keep away from friends who were offending. Although Anna wanted to move area in order to avoid the pressure from friends or family who were offending, she needed to remain in her current tenancy to be near to her looked-after daughter for access reasons. Finally, Vic was conscious of the fact that his current offending was exacerbated by living in a certain housing scheme: 'Most people in [area] have got nothing ... [The area] is a shambles, a pure shambles'.

Many came from families disadvantaged by poverty and *unemployment*. Coupled with the lack of social capital within the family to aid the transition to employment (Allatt and Yeandle, 1992), the vagaries of the youth labour market meant that few of these young people had experienced sustained periods of employment, which often precluded them from spending not only economic but also social and symbolic capital. And yet many of the young people also spoke of their preference for 'honest money' through the legitimate means of employment, and certainly many implied that if they received an income from gainful employment, they had no reason to offend. Pete, for example, felt that unemployment made him vulnerable in terms of re-offending: 'I've got debts with the bank, I've got problems with the Housing ... [but] that's through my own fault. So I'm gonna dig myself out that hole and start again, get a job, get money coming in, get everything paid up and clear myself'.

Involvement in the criminal justice system was an impetus to stopping offending, but also a constraint to sustaining a non-offending lifestyle through legitimate means. Coles (2000) has argued that the youth justice system in particular has a poor track record in preventing further offending amongst young people, with over three-quarters of young male offenders being reconvicted within two years of a custodial sentence. The main problem for the young people in my study was the lack of opportunities for a 'clean slate', exacerbated by having a criminal record and by continued police 'harassment' rather than encouragement in the process of desistance. For example, both Anna and Derek had pending court cases and felt constrained as a result in terms of planning their futures. Three of the male persisters mentioned at interview that they felt the police harassed them on a regular basis, and Derek suggested that his criminal record and pending court cases prevented him from finding a tenancy of his own and a legitimate form of employment.

The concept of social recognition

The above constraints include both structure and agency, not just the agency of the individual young person but, more importantly, the agency of significant others in the young person's life. It has been shown throughout the analysis how important other people are to young people in transition and that young people may resort to crime as one means of attaining reciprocal relations and status with others, whether this be with family members, friends or the wider society. Young people from working class backgrounds are often denied access to social networks as well as to the cultural goods, services and opportunities afforded their more affluent counterparts. As Young (1999: 12) points out in relation to young men:

> [They] are barred from the race-track of the meritocratic society yet remain glued to the television sets and media which alluringly portray the glittering prizes of a wealthy society ... Being denied the respect of others, they create a subculture that revolves around masculine powers and 'respect'.

Young suggests that the 'luck of the draw' mentality in postmodern society – which exemplifies individualism and inequality – is likely to exacerbate criminal activity (ibid.: 198). He stresses the need for reciprocity between the citizen and the state.

According to de Vries (1968: 9) reciprocity is:

> ... a multi-sided active relationship in which the action of any side towards any goal, of itself, promotes and engenders action by the other side towards the same goal ... and all contributions give the participants the conviction of equivalence, and ... are essential to the action of the organism as a whole.

De Vries cites the discipline of philosophy in asserting that 'reciprocal relationships are the only durable, satisfying human relationships' (ibid.: 11), and that limited responsibility and boredom, and the resultant hostility and dissatisfaction generated, are obstacles to such reciprocal arrangements. Likewise, Sennett (2003: 219) argues that mutuality requires recognition in order to make giving and receiving a meaningful exchange, and that 'reciprocity is the foundation of mutual respect'.

The concept of social recognition was described in Chapter 1 as the attainment of a combination of accumulation and expenditure of capital that is durable and legitimated. Social recognition suggests that people both recognize the needs of others (generativity) and are concurrently recognized in addressing those needs (responsibility). It is this 'duality' of recognition that is crucial in ensuring durability and legitimation.

The analysis in this chapter suggests that persisters lacked opportunities for expenditure and experienced more constraints than desisters in the transition to adulthood. The vast majority of these persisters were experiencing structural constraints in their lives at the time of interview and lacked opportunities for expenditure of capital through conventional means. However, those who had stopped offending seemed to have greater opportunities for expenditure of capital and the majority of desisters stated they were *not* experiencing difficulties in their lives currently. Whilst the limits of this secondary analysis are acknowledged, developing this approach could be very fruitful in further understanding and helping to explain the processes of offending and desistance in the transition to adulthood.

Conclusions

Given the large number of young people in this study who had stopped offending before they reached so-called 'adulthood' (10 male and 10 female respondents who had officially stopped offending two years following interview were under the age of 25 (Jones, 1996)), it would seem that offending and desistance are not correlated with 'childhood', 'youth' and 'adulthood' *per se*, but are correlated more with levels of responsibility and legitimacy. Indeed, as highlighted in the previous chapter, the factors most often associated with adulthood – stable employment or one's own home and family – were not achieved in the majority of cases, irrespective of the age at which the respondents stopped offending. This suggests that there are other factors affecting one's propensity or otherwise to stop offending rather than age or adulthood *per se*, and this is where Bourdieu's concept of capital accumulation and its suggested counterpart, expenditure, come to the fore. Whilst many of the desisters were still in the transition phase of youth, they seemed to have already found or been given opportunities to spend as well as accumulate capital. However, from an analysis of the case studies of those still offending, these opportunities seemed at best temporary and at worst non-existent.

Bourdieu (1986: 249–50) has suggested that social capital gained from a network of connections is not 'a natural given ... [but] is the product of an endless effort ... [resulting in] durable obligations subjectively felt (gratitude, respect, friendship) or institutionally guaranteed (rights)'. The importance of other people in the transition to adulthood cannot be underestimated – family in childhood; peers, partners and professional workers in youth; and family, friends, colleagues and partners in adulthood. They all seem to play a role in enabling children and young people not only to accrue but also, as they get older, to spend their various forms of capital.

Being in control is a major influence in one's propensity either to offend or act in a conventional manner. Crime, particularly if successful, can give one the air of being in control (Katz, 1991) and suggests competence (Shover, 1996). In relation to desistance, Maruna (2001) and Burnett (2003) suggest that a feeling of personal agency in one's life is helpful in the desistance process and as Shover and Thompson (1992: 92) point out, a stake in conformity 'improves the odds of desistance'. Accumulating certain types of capital can be relatively easy, although not necessarily via legitimate means. In the liminal phase, limited rights and limited access to mainstream opportunities severely restrict one's access to capital, although class inequalities also tend to restrict access to capital more generally within the population. Without responsibility, rights and opportunities, however, expenditure of capital is difficult to achieve, thus restricting one's access to social recognition.

The processes of offending (for those young people that *do* offend) and transition tend to run parallel courses, based not only on age but also on levels of capital accumulation and expenditure. This parallel course is most apparent for young people from working class backgrounds who have limited access to legitimate capital to ease the transition to adulthood. Both offending and transitions are processes that result from a perceived need by young people to develop, experiment and interact with different people at different phases, and to achieve eventual recognition within the wider society. It has been argued in this chapter that durability and legitimacy, crucial factors in the achievement of social recognition, cannot readily occur during the youth phase, as this phase is seen as transient and lacking in legitimate opportunities for young people. Whilst offending during the youth phase can increase one's short-term accumulation of capital, it is unlikely to address the need for expenditure of capital or for longer-term capital accumulation. However, once young people have access to durable and legitimate opportunities for responsibility taking and generativity, thereby developing opportunities for expenditure of capital as well as accumulation, it is more likely that desistance will occur.

Chapter 8

Conclusions

The transition from family to school along with changes in friendship networks as children move into adolescence seems to be a promising area of exploration for criminologists ... Similarly, learning more about the transitions from adolescence to adulthood is critical for understanding the development of social ties in adulthood.

(Sampson and Laub, 1993: 250)

... it would be difficult to comprehend an individual criminal career without also considering concurrent, wider experiences of transition not normally surveyed in criminology.

(MacDonald and Marsh, 2005: 172)

You know how your life goes through all these stages ... your teens, you're a bit young and stupid, but in your twenties, you start to think a wee bit more about life and the person who you are, trying to get a wee bit of identity yourself and trying to better yourself in some way ... trying to get more intelligent.

(Vicky, 27)

Introduction

The aims of this book have been to examine the process of offending from the perspective of young people and to look for parallels in the reasons given for onset and desistance. In so doing, the research drew comparisons between the three phases of offending (onset, maintenance and desistance) and the three phases of youth transition (childhood, youth and adulthood). It revealed that offending may well have been either masking or manifesting other problems in young people's lives, and could have demonstrated a need for, rather than a rebellion against, social integration.

Whilst the majority of the sample were high-tariff offenders (having received intensive probation in the past), their offending overall was not 'serious' but predominantly involved theft, possession of drugs and assault. The young people in this study were working class, disadvantaged and generally adversely affected by family upheaval, by a lack of stability and continuity in childhood and by limited opportunities for love, attention and encouragement in the transition to adulthood. The majority tended to start offending as a means of social integration (through impressing their friends or acquiring consumer goods), although a small minority suggested more personal factors such as rebellion against a traumatic childhood or as a means of relieving boredom. The majority of these young people were currently or previously experiencing situations of discontinuity, instability and liminality. Many spoke of their childhoods in terms of moving home area, living with differing family members, living with mothers who had several changes of partner and being looked after in residential care. Not only did variable levels of consistency and stability in their families and communities restrict their sources of capital, it also undermined their attempts to accumulate such capital through relatively stable friendship groups. It could be argued that this variable access to significant others both heightened their perceived need to buy their friends when such opportunities presented themselves and to fit into such friendship circles in the time allowed. Offending was, to many, an obvious vehicle in the rush to make and keep friends. The social recognition gained from peers was crucial at a time when other people and situations in their lives were in a state of flux and uncertainty.

The limitations of current theory

Many theories of offending and desistance have elements which, when combined with other perspectives, have proved useful in informing the analysis within this book. The interactive emphasis of subcultural theory, coupled with the structural inequalities implied by strain theory, are helpful in explaining why young people tend to start offending in late childhood, in the company of their peers, and why they tend to offend for monetary or sociability reasons. Matza's theory of drift (1964) and differential association (Sutherland and Cressey, 1970; 1978) provide a useful framework for understanding the temporary and intermittent nature of youth offending throughout the process from onset to desistance, although these theories have shortcomings in terms of being able to explain why many young people make a conscious decision to desist from offending through proactively breaking away from their immediate circle of friends.

Nevertheless, Chapter 2 revealed that there are few criminological theories which can account not only for the three phases of offending in parallel but also for 'false positives' – those individuals who desist from crime against all (academic) expectations. In terms of incorporating the three phases of offending within theories, this book has shown that these young people's early offending behaviour was often an interactive and group activity, but their later offending tended to be a solitary and expedient activity for monetary gain. However, whilst their experiences of offending may mirror those of the majority of young offenders in the Western world, their experiences do not necessarily mirror the criminological theories designed to explain them. Subcultural theory may be relevant to the onset of offending, in that young people tend to congregate in groups and gain identity through that interaction, but it cannot readily account for the solitary nature of the maintenance phase of offending or indeed for desistance. Equally, labelling theory may prove relevant to much offending in the maintenance phase, but cannot easily account for onset. Feminist theories are better able to explain the different treatment of young women in the criminal justice system but are less able to account for the divergent reasons given for offending by young men and women as they move from the onset to the maintenance phase.

In terms of 'false positives', labelling, social control, subcultural and strain theories, for example, have been criticized for not being able to account for desistance which occurs without any concurrent and obvious changes in structural circumstances. For example, individuals desist from crime without gaining employment, a stable income or a family of their own. Many of the young people in this sample also managed to stop offending, not only in times of poverty and addiction, but also in the face of continued harassment by, for example, the police or the 'subcultural' milieu of their offending peers. Thus, whilst still labelled as offenders within their communities, they nevertheless managed to desist from crime. Although theories of desistance have explored the type and quality of turning points in young people's lives which may enable desistance to occur, none have systematically explored the institutional factors that inhibit or enhance capital accumulation and expenditure, factors which may well affect one's propensity to offend and one's opportunities for social recognition.

Applying the concept of capital to youth transitions

Bourdieu's concept of capital has proved to be crucial in linking the phases of transition with those of offending. The period of youth is one where boundaries are blurred, guidance and support are often reduced or passing from one source (the family) to another (the friendship group), and responsibilities are not wholly acknowledged as legitimate or sustainable. Offending in the transition to adulthood is one readily accessible vehicle that disadvantaged young people can use to move from the relative shelter of the family, through the vagaries of youth, to emerge at the ultimate point of societal acceptance, integration and belonging. In other words, offending is a strategy, however temporary or misguided, that young people can adopt to achieve social, economic, cultural or symbolic capital. Between childhood and adulthood, young people from disadvantaged backgrounds have few socially recognized means of legitimating their stake in the social world but may see offending or its benefits as their only means of gaining recognition meantime, even if such recognition only comes from their friends.

In early youth, offending and the resultant attention or influence of friends may provide crucial sources of capital for these young people, during a time when they possibly lack attention, protection or encouragement from family or the wider community. Although the family can be a renewed and enduring source of support and social capital for young people as they get older, it seems the case that in the youth phase, the friendship group takes precedence over the family as a means of consolidating and reinforcing one's own identity within a social setting. In early adulthood, however, the criminal justice system tended to erode what little capital accumulation had been gained from offending or indeed from conventional activities or relationships in the past. Nevertheless, once outside the criminal justice system, these young people were more likely to be able to accumulate and retain capital with opportunities for renewed family contact, relationships with conventional partners, employment and responsibility. However, what is missing from this analysis is the answer to the question of how capital in its various forms can reduce the likelihood of offending when such capital can be gained from offending itself. The answer, I argue, lies in the concept of social recognition, where a combination of expenditure and accumulation of capital that is durable and legitimate eases both the transition to adulthood and the transition to desistance.

The importance of social recognition

Social recognition has been defined as the attainment of a durable and legitimate combination of capital accumulation and expenditure. This book argues that only with that combination of capital accumulation and expenditure, in a reciprocal and durable dialogue with others, are individuals and groups able to fully reap the benefits of social, economic, cultural and symbolic capital, and thus gain access to wider social recognition. Such recognition comes over time: in Bourdieu's language, it is the durability and legitimacy of the capital (its *sustainability* and *social credibility* over time) that creates social recognition. However, for children and young people durability and legitimacy of capital are rarely possible within the liminal phase of transition, and such capital can only be sustained within the relative stability of adulthood, when greater opportunities for expenditure as well as accumulation are available to them. This accords with Willis's (1990: 7) suggestion that youth culture more generally (and this could be seen to include offending behaviour) has often provided a vehicle towards self and social identity for young people in transition:

> ... the teenage and early adult years are important ... because it is here ... where people are formed most self-consciously through their own symbolic and other activities ... through which they understand themselves and their possibilities for the rest of their lives.

As noted in Chapter 7, the analysis of capital accumulation and expenditure in relation to these young people suggests that the persisters lacked opportunities for expenditure of their capital through conventional means and experienced more constraints than desisters in the transition to adulthood. Desistance did not come with age *per se* for these young people, but with increased opportunities to spend capital through generativity and responsibility taking. The women in this respect seemed more likely to respond to the accumulation and expenditure of social capital (given their emphasis on relational factors) whereas the men continued to seek symbolic capital but were frustrated in this as a result of structural constraints. The women also seemed to have greater access to opportunities to both accumulate and spend capital through conventional means as they grew older. For example, the women were more than twice as likely as the men to have children of their own and their own tenancy. The women were also more likely to have access to formal (professional) or informal (personal) support mechanisms in addressing offending or drug and alcohol problems. Because of the women's more collective and emotional approach, other people were the most likely recipients of these women's expenditure of capital through generativity and responsibilities as mothers or partners, thereby enhancing their social recognition. The men, on the other hand, being more separatist and individual, tended to have fewer opportunities for generativity and responsibility, thus reducing their opportunities for social recognition through relational means. This could be a reason why the young women's offending was generally more short-term and less serious than the men's.

The concepts of capital accumulation and expenditure can contribute towards an understanding of the timing of onset, maintenance and desistance as well as gender differences, and it is argued here that these concepts are more helpful in this understanding than age, agency or structure in isolation. Accumulation of capital requires, to a certain extent, both responsibilities and access to opportunities; however, children and young people rarely have such opportunities because of their status as 'liminal entities' (Turner, 1969), not least those from a working class background. Jenkins (2003, pers. comm.) has described Bourdieu's concepts of social, economic, cultural and symbolic capital as 'imprecise heuristic devices', but their imprecision has enabled greater scope for appropriation and adaptation within this book, and in so doing, has allowed for a fuller understanding of both youth transitions and youth offending as processes of change.

Developing the concept of social recognition

The opening quotations to this chapter provide clues for further studies of young offenders' experiences of the transition to adulthood. These could include an exploration of their preferences and opportunities for responsibility taking and generativity throughout childhood and youth, as well as the timing of such activity in relation to their offending during those transitional periods. However, social recognition is not a concept easily amenable to operationalism. Certain factors associated with social recognition may be subjected to more quantitative investigation. For example, one could identify factors likely to create opportunities for capital accumulation and expenditure (along the lines of Tables 3.1 and 7.1), as well as factors likely to restrict such opportunities (as per Figure 7.1). Equally, factors associated specifically with capital expenditure (e.g. generativity and responsibility taking) versus capital accumulation could be compared with levels of offending over time for specific groups of people. It would be informative to analyse the offending pattern over time of young carers, for example, who may score highly on capital expenditure, have few opportunities for capital accumulation and have little durability or legitimacy of capital accruing from their caring role. Although many offenders talk of restitution to society once they have stopped offending, it may be worth examining the extent to which generativity is rehabilitative for the individual as a result of shame or guilt or whether it is more of a pragmatic desire to give of one's own experiences in preventing similar problems for others. Certainly this research suggested the latter.

From an international perspective, further research into the differing lengths and qualities of transitions in varying countries compared with those countries' youth offending rates may also shed some light on whether youth transitions *per se* (i.e. across cultures) have a specific effect on offending behaviour. The criminalization of the young indigenous populations of Australia and New Zealand and the low youth crime rates in Japan would warrant further attention from a social recognition perspective. Whether the findings from this study could be replicated in other cultures remains to be seen, but the concept of social recognition offers a potential tool for examining offending amongst other youth populations in other transitional arrangements. It also offers the potential to explain onset, maintenance and desistance through an analysis of the formal and informal social bonds and opportunities for expenditure versus accumulation of capital over time.

To conclude, this research aimed to further the debate about the causes and correlates of youth offending and desistance. The voices of the young people in this book, their experiences of marginalization and their expressed desire for integration and conventionality led to the concepts of capital accumulation and expenditure, and from there to the concept of social recognition. The study explored both young people's experiences of offending as a process of change and the potential of Bourdieu's concepts of capital as a tool to link the phases of offending with those of youth transition. Social recognition is a concept that may further an understanding of youth offending and exemplify young people's wish for legitimate and sustained opportunities within the wider society. The concept of social recognition highlights the need for reciprocity, in that the wider society also needs to demonstrate the value it places on young people's capacities and responsibilities in the transition to adulthood. Until there is a reciprocal and constructive approach taken by society to the problems faced by its young people in transition, then a greater understanding of youth offending will continue to elude us. The young people in this book demonstrated a strong desire for integration, interdependence, responsibility and trust, and they looked in part to adults to give them that sense of social recognition. Gillian (aged 29) expressed it thus at the end of her interview: 'Put faith in me. Give me another chance. Trust me.' Such a plea, if heard, could go a long way to alleviating the problems for young people in transition, and in so doing, could well reduce the demands made on the youth and criminal justice systems.

Appendixes

APPENDIX A: METHODOLOGY

Introduction

Much youth research until recent years focused on the problems rather than the potential of young people (Barry, 2005; Miles, 2000). Such theories also tended to focus on young men rather than young women (Gelsthorpe and Morris, 1990) and to stress subcultural idiosyncracies rather than mainstream norms. Young people had become passive victims of structural imbalances within society, rather than active negotiators within their social worlds, or alternatively, they had become manipulative actors rationally circumventing structural forces. Sociologists of youth tended to position themselves on either the structure side or the agency side, but not to straddle both. More recently, there has been a greater awareness of the two-way relationship between, on the one hand, structural opportunities and constraints and, on the other hand, young people's ability to construct their own identities (Miles, 2000). Miles argues that 'this divide has served to undermine the development of an effective sociology of youth which will only emerge when cultural aspects of young people's lives are considered in the situated context of structural constraints and vice versa' (ibid.: 35). Not only have young people been set apart in terms of their behaviour, but also in terms of their views. According to Miles (2000: 6), the sociology of subculture and the sociology of youth transitions failed until recently 'to accommodate actors' own accounts or experiences', although, amongst others, Becker (1963), Hall and Jefferson (1976) and Willis (1977) in the 1960s and 1970s argued for actors' narratives to be taken into account.

These developments are part of a general social scientific dilemma over whether people should be studied as 'subjects' or as 'objects'. The latter approach is exemplified by the positivist school, which suggests that people could be studied as the object of enquiry, and that only observable facts are valid. However, there is increasing importance being placed on 'listening' – whether this be to the consumer in the market place, to the patient in health care or to the client in social work: even when exposed to the same structural constraints, people will react differently, thus suggesting that a sociogenic approach does not allow for individual narratives (Bryman, 1988; Leibrich, 1993). For these narratives to be incorporated, a phenomenological approach is required in conjunction with a sociogenic one (Maruna, 2001).

It is a relatively new phenomenon, emanating from the 1980s, that service users, and in particular offenders, have been asked their views about the service they receive (Barry, 2000). But young offenders are rarely seen as 'service users' *per se*, and are thus less likely to be asked about their views not just about a particular 'service' they receive, but more importantly, about why they think they became involved in offending in the first place, what they thought about their behaviour and how, if at all, they managed to stop offending. This study aimed to confront these issues by engaging in direct discussion with young people who had offended in the past and to seek their views and advice about the nature of their offending and its advantages and disadvantages over time.

The rationale for the methods used

The research questions for this study were as follows:

- What are young people's experiences and views of starting, continuing and stopping offending?
- Is there a relationship between young people's reasons for starting, continuing and stopping offending?
- Are there gender differences in the reasons young people give for starting, continuing and stopping offending?

Butters (1976: 259) suggests that a flexible approach is important in fieldwork, one that allows modifications based on respondents' views: 'the focus and strategy of the fieldwork must be evolved through ... attentiveness to hosts' accounts of what in their situations is problematic to them'. As I was interested in young people's perceptions of their social networks, support networks and attitudes to offending and conformity, I decided that this type of subjective information was better obtained through in-depth interviews rather than, for example, closed or multiple-choice questions within a questionnaire format. In order to examine the research questions more fully, I was particularly keen to speak to those young people who had stopped offending but who had been persistent offenders in the past, the persistency element allowing for a starker contrast to be established between the three phases of offending, onset, maintenance and desistance. Because I was interested in any possible continuity between these phases, I decided that there should also be continuity in the sample, thus asking the *same* respondents to talk about the three phases in parallel. I also wanted to speak to individuals aged 18 to 30, since at the lower end (18), persisters would be more likely to be included, and at the upper end (30), not only would it be reasonable to expect relatively accurate memory recall but also desistance and the 'transition to adulthood' are more likely to have occurred.

Accessing the sample

Given the inherent difficulties in accessing young offenders, a sample of 40 was deemed to be large enough to enable the collection of enough quantitative data to make basic numerical comparison feasible, whilst also offering a wide enough but manageable range of experiences and views within a qualitative framework. This sample size is also broadly consistent with the widely-held convention in social research that more than 20 qualitative interviews within a sub-sample is likely to be subject to the 'law of diminishing returns', i.e. few new insights are revealed from additional cases. This generally proved to be the case with this sample.

After attempting to access young offenders via the police and social work departments, which was virtually impossible because of the requirements of the Data Protection Act (1998) amongst other factors, it was decided to use a purposive sampling method to gain access to potential respondents via a national voluntary organization, and to augment this with snowballing techniques if necessary. This organization ran intensive probation projects in various areas of Scotland, all of which had come into operation between 1990 and 1995. They agreed to my accessing a sample through several of their projects, on the condition that I added an additional question in the interview schedule about the effectiveness or otherwise of intensive probation and undertook to provide feedback to the organization about the overall research findings. It appeared feasible, given the numbers of clients being referred to this organization throughout its projects in Scotland, that I would be able to gain access to the desired total of 40 previously persistent offenders, although not necessarily an equal gender mix, since the numbers of women referred were very low (see below).

Initial contact was made in 1999 through project staff to former clients of the four intensive probation projects identified by the voluntary organization. Lists were drawn up by project staff of all young people who had been given a court order on or before 30 June 1997, with intensive probation as a condition. This date was at least two years before starting access negotiations, so as to allow a potential two-year period to have elapsed between being an 'active' client and being interviewed for this study. However, it is acknowledged that I could not expect such clients to have necessarily stopped offending during that two-year period. Letters and consent forms from project staff were sent to potential respondents using either an opt-in or opt-out approach, depending on differing practices in relation to the Data Protection Act. Given the transient and somewhat chaotic lifestyle of many known offenders, an 'opt-out' approach is often the most preferable means for researchers of contacting potential respondents, leaving the onus on the researcher to contact the client rather than vice versa, not least if the client has not been in touch with the referring organization for some years, as was the case with some of this sample.

Appropriate respondents were then approached by myself, following an agreed cut-off date for returns of consent forms, and given further information about the research prior to choosing whether or not to participate in the study. Of the 23 ex-clients contacted via the means of an opt-in letter, only five replied, and these five were subsequently interviewed (two men and three women). The opt-out letter was sent to approximately 85 ex-clients (only four of whom were women). All four women were interviewed, and 19 men were interviewed from this latter source (one of whom was subsequently withdrawn because he was a one-off offender). Through this voluntary organization, therefore, I had gained interviews with 20 young men and seven young women. Snowballing was used to boost this female sample in one instance, where one young woman's friend had not returned the reply slip to the voluntary organization, but subsequently agreed to participate in the research. I wanted an equal number of male to female respondents so as to be able to draw comparisons between the two sexes, and so as to avoid the criticism that young women tend to have 'occasional walk on parts' in criminological studies of this kind (Scraton, 1990: 18). I thus managed to boost the female sample, again purposively, via additional approaches to several social work departments and other organizations working in the offender field. These contacts were informally arranged and led to social workers identifying young women who met the criteria (in terms of age and probation experience, so as to at least partly match the men in the sample in terms of previous disposals). It was thus possible to gain a sample of 20 male and 20 female respondents, aged between 18 and 33, all of whom had previous experience of probation, but could not otherwise be matched in terms of level and seriousness of offending over time. In all, the time period from starting negotiations with various agencies for access to a sample, and completing the fieldwork, was approximately 19 months, on a part-time basis. The fieldwork began in February 2000 and was completed in April 2001. Interviews were transcribed throughout the fieldwork period.

The difficulties faced in attempting to access a sample of 40 young offenders, with an equal sex ratio, should not be underestimated, not least with the increasing constraints placed on researchers by data protection legislation. It requires diplomacy with gatekeepers, a keen awareness of the ethical considerations, and perhaps most importantly, a level of persistence in tracking down young people whose movements tend to be both uncertain and covert. In addition, young female offenders are less accessible through intensive probation projects, partly because they are less persistent overall in their offending compared to young men, partly because such projects cannot offer a 'women-only' service[1] and partly because women's persistence in offending is often related to drug problems which are better dealt with by alternative disposals (Sommers *et al.*, 1994; McLennan, 2003, pers. comm.).

The advantages of accessing a sample through an intensive probation agency are a) that one can be sure that they were *either* persistent offenders *or* had committed at least one serious offence, since intensive probation is a 'high-tariff' disposal; and b) the intensive probation project can act as 'gatekeeper' in terms of identifying suitable candidates from their records and making the initial contact on behalf of the researcher. The disadvantages of this method of accessing a sample are a) that the researcher is, to a greater or lesser degree, dependent on the said gatekeeper for access (hence the problem of gaining a sample of 40 via this means); b) there is no way of gauging whether clients have actually desisted until contact has been made (although I was fortunate in gaining a relatively evenly balanced sample of persisters and desisters); and c) I could not get an even number of male and female respondents (the projects catered almost exclusively for men) or young people from ethnic minority backgrounds (all bar one of the sample were white European, with one Afro-Caribbean young woman). However, in respect of this sample, the attrition rate was fortunately very low: I was unsuccessful in tracing only eight young people, whilst a further three declined to be interviewed, mainly because of other commitments.

Issues of sample representativeness

Much criminological research uses incarcerated individuals as sample respondents, partly because such offenders are readily accessible. Given that to be incarcerated one has to be detected, that only one in three crimes is reported to the police, that only one in ten crimes results in prosecution and that under 14 per cent of all persons with a charge proved in Scotland in 2001 received a custodial sentence, it is doubtful whether many of these criminological research studies can claim representativeness in their sampling methods. Interviewing young people in prison would have been a more convenient way of accessing a sample, but that would not have allowed me to sample desisters as well as persisters, nor to interview young people in a neutral and 'safe' setting that might ensure confidentiality, openness and trust: crucial factors when undertaking sensitive qualitative research with young offenders.

Some critics of traditional criminological studies have suggested that many community-based samples identified in such studies (for example, male, teenage, less serious and less persistent offenders) do not depict the 'average' offender – another reason, perhaps, why some studies try to deflect such criticism by interviewing older, incarcerated respondents. I have addressed this potential criticism by accessing the majority of individuals in this study through an intensive probation project. Such projects have strict guidelines on who is appropriate for an Intensive Probation Order, in terms of persistence and seriousness of offending; as a result, referring agencies, sheriffs and project staff alike have rigorous mechanisms in place for ensuring that no young person is 'up-tariffed' as a result of being given such an Order.

From the list of offences mentioned by the young people in this research (see Appendix B), it can be seen that the majority of the sample's offences, whilst more serious and persistent than the national picture for offending in Scotland (Scottish Executive, 2002), were generally unsophisticated in nature, for example breach of the peace, shoplifting and possession of drugs. Figures for Scotland suggest that under 4 per cent of all crimes and offences committed by 16–30-year-olds in 2001 were serious offences (e.g. homicide, robbery and serious assault). however, the type and frequency of offences for this sample of young people seem to be well above the national average for current young offenders in Scotland (Scottish Executive, 2002), given that their offences include attempted murder, serious assault, police assault and robbery.

The interview process

The interview schedule developed as a result of my interest not only in compiling demographic and offending histories, but also in developing a dialogue with respondents regarding the processes they went through in starting, continuing and stopping offending. Both the vulnerabilities (in age, background and behaviour) of the group under study and the complexities inherent in making sense of crime and criminality suggested that a discursive, informal interview was the best medium through which to engage with this sample. A qualitative interview of this nature can also be a cathartic experience. Talking about certain aspects of one's life in detail is something that many young people have rarely had the opportunity to do (Barry, 2001a). As one young woman in the current study stated at the end of the interview: 'It's good to talk about it. It helps talking about things, you know ... 'Cos you're not bottling it up inside' (Anna, 21). This view was matched by a young man in a previous study I undertook of children's experiences of growing up: 'nobody's ever done that, sat down and just talked ... about my life' (Barry, 2001a: 34). Equally, young offenders rarely have the opportunity to analyse their experiences of offending with anyone other than a social worker and for reasons other than those pertaining to punishment or rehabilitation, and in this respect, talking to a neutral third party may have motivated them to be perhaps more enthusiastic and frank than usual.

A total of 43 interviews were undertaken, although three of these were subsequently not used because they did not fully fit the criteria (two of these respondents were first-time offenders and the third had only offended marginally in adolescence). Two pilot interviews, which were subsequently incorporated into the total number of 40 interviews, enabled me to 'test out' my line of questioning, to iron out any stylistic or linguistic problems and to monitor the flow and general logic of the schedule. At the start of the interview, I asked these two respondents to give me the additional help and feedback on how to make the interview a meaningful, clear and 'user-friendly' experience for research participants. Their help in this was invaluable whilst not detracting from the overall integrity of the research, since they were asked the same questions as the other respondents, with only slight changes to wording being made as a result of their suggestions.

Three-quarters of the interviews were conducted in respondents' own homes, with four respondents being interviewed in either the project's offices or other agency premises and six being interviewed in prison. In the vast majority of cases, the interview was conducted in a quiet room (even within some of the prisons), usually with no other people present or within earshot, thus limiting the likelihood of interview site bias on the data obtained. However, on some occasions, babies or young children were present during interviews in people's homes. My only reservation about this was where I was concerned that the child might understand some of what was being said – in terms of offending or drug-taking, for example, by the mother – but I either took the lead from the respondent on this or we 'veiled' our conversation where necessary.

The interview lasted on average one and a half hours, and was tape-recorded with the respondent's agreement.[2] It should be pointed out that although dialects varied considerably between the geographical areas under study, and although the transcripts adopted the vernacular language of the respondents, it was nevertheless decided to 'anglicize' the quotations where necessary, partly for ease of understanding by the reader and partly because of the difficulties inherent in phonetically transcribing differing modes of speech.

It was deemed important in my initial negotiation with potential interviewees and in the introduction to these particular interviews to be clear and honest about my intentions for the research and to say what help I wanted from them and why. The first part of the interview was to seek predominantly factual information rather than opinion and to give the respondents time to familiarize themselves with the interviewer and to adjust to the interview environment. This first phase of the interview elicited information such as living arrangements, family status and experiences and perceptions of education and employment.

The subsequent phase of the interview was more in-depth and semi-structured in nature, during which their perceptions were sought about the following issues:

- definitions of offending;
- type and frequency of offending since onset;
- reasons and circumstances surrounding starting, continuing and stopping offending;
- the advantages and disadvantages of starting, continuing and stopping offending;
- factors which helped or hindered the process of starting, continuing and stopping offending;
- future aspirations;
- the effects of outside factors, such as family or significant events, on their pattern of offending.

In order to make the interview process as interesting and engaging as possible for the respondents, four exercises were used (written exercises, graphs and statement cards to illustrate points during the interview), which helped stimulate memory recall, avoid monotony and encourage dialogue. The first of these was a timeline of the type and number of offences committed since childhood and the broadly estimated proportion of times that these offences were detected by the police. The second was grouping their offences on cards, in a way that made sense to them (e.g. 'for money/for fun', 'serious/not serious', etc.), thus eliciting their categorizations of offences and possible rationale for committing them. The third exercise was a graph of levels of involvement in offending (low, medium and high) from the age they started to the present day, which mirrored the first exercise in terms of frequency. The final exercise was another timeline of people and events since childhood that the respondents thought had an impact on their behaviour or attitudes over the years, notably in relation to offending.

The vast majority of these interviews consisted of full and frank discussions about respondents' offending, their childhood experiences and their future aspirations. Interviewing young people in their own homes, where they are in familiar surroundings, helps to break down any barriers between the interviewer and the interviewee. Many had made the effort, in advance of our meeting, to prepare either themselves (for example, by getting up and getting dressed for a morning appointment) or their homes (for example, by tidying up or preparing tea and biscuits). I stressed at the outset of the interview that I wanted their advice rather than to 'interview' them as such, and that they should feel free to 'show me the door' at any point during our discussion, should they so wish. Although I was more interested in their views than they were in mine, I was nevertheless as open and honest when asked for my own opinion as I hope they were with me. This mutual respect and rapport seemed, sadly, to be rare for them in their dealings with 'older' 'professionals'. During the interview, I often helped make tea, or played with a child, so as to ease the pressure on the respondent or to demonstrate my gratitude for their time and hospitality.[3] I am sure that this interactive and relaxed approach greatly enhanced the quality of the interviews overall.

Ethics

It is becoming increasingly difficult for researchers to retain freedom of access within the research process because of, in particular, the Data Protection Act (1998), which has justifiably curtailed the activities of researchers in choosing who, where and why to interview. For these reasons, most research organizations follow a certain code of ethics in social science research and in this study various codes of ethics were consulted, in particular, the codes of research ethics from the University of Stirling and the British Sociological Association (1996). Such codes of ethics tend to be subsumed under the following three headings: informed consent, minimization of harm and confidentiality/anonymity.

Informed consent

Informed consent refers not only to the need to give respondents an honest and full account of the aims of the research but also the need to ensure that they do not feel pressurized into participating.

If respondents feel they are a part of and fully informed about the research aims, they are more likely to be honest and constructive in their comments. Therefore, at the start of the interview I informed the young people about the reasons for, and methods used in, undertaking the research and what was requested of them as respondents. This included why I wanted to speak with them, how I had identified them, that I wanted to tape our conversation, how I would use quotations and what I intended to do with the final report. We both signed a written agreement, or 'contract' at the start of the interview and each respondent was given the right to withdraw from the process at any time during the interview, although none did.

Minimization of harm

In any research study, it is always important to ensure that nobody is personally harmed by the research process or its findings. However, where research is studying former or current offenders, it is even more important to respect and protect respondents' rights to anonymity and control over the use of the data. One controversial exception to this rule may be in situations where information is divulged to the researcher that may harm the respondent or other people, i.e. disclosure of abuse.

In this study, each respondent was initially told that it was their prerogative whether or not to divulge information, and that if I were to ask them something which they would rather not answer, then to tell me so. I attempted to reassure them that I would not press them for information that might either incriminate or upset them. In expanding on this issue, I stressed that they should not divulge any planned offence or any undetected but identifiable previous offence, as this would put both me and the respondent in an awkward position. I took my lead in this respect from Leibrich's (1992) study, and informed participants that they could tell me in confidence that they had robbed a bank yesterday, but not to tell me *which* bank. However, they should not tell me if they planned to rob the Bank of Scotland in the High Street tomorrow, as I would feel morally compelled to warn those potentially affected. Taking this approach leaves the ball firmly in the court of the respondent and it is therefore difficult to gauge if information was withheld from me as a result.

Wary of the potential harm to participants of talking about upsetting events in the past, I was prepared to offer advice to the young people involved, after the interview was completed, in relation to relevant help or advice from other agencies or individuals. Nevertheless, none of the respondents seemed, or suggested that they were, upset by the interview itself. However, I always purposefully ended the interview by talking about their past achievements and future aspirations, which was generally seen as very much a positive conclusion to the interview process.

Confidentiality and anonymity

Respondents were informed that any law-breaking activity they had done in the past and which they shared with me would remain confidential (albeit with the proviso discussed in the 'Minimization of harm' section above). The respondents were also assured that, like it or not, they were 'a number' rather than a name and their identity would be withheld in the final report. Both myself and the respondent signed a contract to this effect.

Lists of the potential sample population and subsequent transcripts and other identifying information were kept in a locked cupboard. The typist who transcribed the interviews was known to, and trusted by, me and all names and places were deleted from the transcripts prior to inputting the data onto the qualitative data analysis package Nud*ist and the statistical analysis package SPSS. The interviews were numbered 1–43[4] and where young people are quoted directly in this report, each quotation is identified only by a pseudonym and the age of the speaker.

Reconviction data

Accessing reconviction data was intended to complement the respondents' own memories of offence types and frequency. Self-report data on offending *on their own* can often be unreliable for several reasons. Such data can be affected by poor respondent recall, are dependent upon an open and honest perspective by the respondent and may be influenced by the respondent's rapport with the researcher. Farrall and Bowling suggest that personal narratives may be biased, however inadvertently: 'respondents may attempt to imbue their previous lives with rationality and intent' (Farrall and Bowling, 1997: 13).

So as to minimize the impact of bias in a researcher/respondent interaction, supplementing the data with official reconviction data can, to a certain extent, act as a triangulation[5] method of ensuring more accurate data collection. To this end, reconviction data were sought towards the end of the fieldwork period with the permission of respondents and via the auspices of the various social work departments involved. At the end of the interview, each respondent signed a consent form agreeing to my accessing their previous convictions data. No one refused permission for access to this information. In accessing these data, it was necessary to first approach social work departments for SCRO numbers. Relevant social work departments were given a copy of the respondents' consent forms with client details and once the SCRO numbers were collected, these were sent in an anonymized form to the Criminal Justice Statistics Branch of the Scottish Executive to access the reconviction data. These data covered all criminal convictions from the age of 16 (and often those offences dealt with by the children's hearings system prior to the age of 16) until September, 2002, 17–31 months following interview, depending on the time of interview.

Categorizing and interpreting the data

Categorizing unstructured qualitative data can often undermine the very reason why such a data collection approach was adopted in the first place (Jones, 1985), in that the researcher's categorization can predetermine the resultant interpretation of the text. However, to do otherwise would be to leave the data in too unstructured and diverse a form to allow any subsequent meaningful interpretation and explanation.

With the help of the data analysis package, Nud*ist, I started analysis by categorizing the data by the questions asked in the interview schedule, resulting in broad headings such as demographic details; starting, continuing and stopping offending; and perceptions of change, the future, offending generally and the criminal justice system. Further categories arose from these findings: for example, drugs and alcohol, maturation, realization and supportive factors. Because the sample number was relatively manageable and because I wanted to familiarize myself as much as possible with each transcription as an entity in its own right, I did not use Nud*ist to its full capacity. Equally, whilst I entered much of the quantitative data onto SPSS, this data package only served to calculate aggregate numbers and was not used in a more sophisticated fashion.

From the data on reasons for, influences in and advantages and disadvantages of starting, continuing and stopping offending, four key organizational categories emerged that were common to each phase of offending. These were: practical, personal, relational and monetary, and it was felt that Bourdieu's four types of capital – social, economic, cultural and symbolic – matched the four organizational categories that were used to make sense of the original data, and also offered a bridge between both the offending phases and the phases of transition. I was concerned, though, not to pre-empt the findings from the discussions with young people since this was primarily an exploratory study; their views and experiences led me to a secondary analysis of the data using Bourdieu's concepts of capital.

Analytical considerations

In undertaking this study, I wanted to explore further the anomaly between, on the one hand, what the literature suggests are the opportunities that promote desistance and, on the other hand, the fact that many offenders desist from crime without having acquired any of these opportunities. Equally, what are the differences in young people's explanations for why they start and stop offending? I was also interested to see whether acquiring responsibilities or a 'different' persona in adulthood was in any way connected to the process of desistance. Whilst these issues were not specifically explored at interview, the wording of the interview schedule was such as to enable these issues to emerge if and when appropriate.

The secondary analysis for this study took place *as a result of* the findings from the primary analysis of the respondents' experiences of starting and stopping offending. I should explain why I found Bourdieu's concepts more useful in my secondary analysis than, for example, those of Giddens (1976; 1979; 1984; 1991), even though Giddens's work has attracted more attention than that of Bourdieu in criminological circles (see, for example, Smith, 1986; Bottoms, 1993; Bottoms and Wiles, 1992; Farrall and Bowling, 1999). Giddens (1984) sees equality as being resolved by social inclusion of individuals into the status quo, tending thus to ignore class-based inequalities. Giddens promotes the ethos of active citizenship where rights and responsibilities go hand-in-hand. He suggests that individualized inequalities can be overcome given that power is an attainable asset to every individual, not just a few. In other words, power need not be 'zero sum'[6] (Haugaard, 2002: 150); thus, 'nobody is completely powerless' (Craib, 1992: 115). Bourdieu, on the other hand, is concerned with structural insecurity rather than with individual risk. He argues that power is indeed a restricted, zero sum resource and that inequalities are collective issues that are class-based rather than personal issues (Callinicos, 1999).

Whilst both Giddens and Bourdieu argue for a 'middle ground' approach to the dichotomy between structure and agency, Giddens's theory of structuration is less concerned about the uneven distribution of power and agency and tends to play down the capacity of individuals over the lifecourse both *'to structure* and avoid *being structured'* (Farrall and Bowling, 1999: 256, emphases in original). Bourdieu, on the other hand, emphasizes the fluid and contextual nature of social action, notably in the constant accumulation and reciprocal appropriation of capital and in the interplay of time and space with the habitus and fields of power. Coupled with his emphasis on structural inequalities, Bourdieu's concepts of capital were also innovative in the criminological field and helped me to compare offending with youth transitions, both of which are dynamic processes of continuity and change within a changing socio-structural environment.

APPENDIX B: CHARACTERISTICS OF THE SAMPLE

Table B.1 Offending histories of respondents

Respondent	Age at interview	Age started offending	Age stopped offending[1]	Length of offending history	No. of previous offences	No. of previous convictions
Males:						
Alec	28	15	24	9	23	11
Bob	20	17	N/A	5+	53	30
Charlie	21	15	20	5	30	21
Derek	21	12	22	10	32	19
Eric	21	13	N/A	10+	72	40
Frank	22	12	23	11	30	14
Graham	21	13	22	9	44	33
Harry	26	13	22	9	38	29
John	23	12	N/A	13+	54	40
Kevin	23	15	N/A	10+	35	21
Len	26	8	N/A	20+	81	47
Martin	24	18	24	6	18	11
Nick	28	8	N/A	20+	51	24
Owen	18	11	N/A	9+	14	9
Pete	19	10	19	9	22	12
David	20	12	N/A	10+	30	18
Rory	23	12	20	8	29	22
Sam	23	15	23	8	28	17
Tom	19	11	20	9	14	11
Vic	23	8	24	16	67	46
Females:						
Laura	27	12	25	13	46	24
Anna	21	14	22	8	38	25
Karen	28	21	29	8	26	14
Bernadette	23	14	21	7	4	4
Diane	21	9	20	11	8	5
Marie	21	15	22	7	20	15
Nina	23	14	24	10	43	18
Alison	20	12	N/A	10+	79	47
Paula	27	19	N/A	10+	15	9
Janet	21	8	16	8	3	2
Carol	29	12	29	17	3	3
Helen	20	10	19	9	15	13
Sarah	27	16	N/A	13+	15	9
Gillian	29	17	N/A	14+	8	4
Vicky	27	22	26	4	5	4
Rhona	22	9	N/A	15+	24	15
Theresa	33	12	31	19	19	12
Cathy	23	17	24	7	25	18
Avril	18	11	17	6	5	3
Yvonne	25	13	24	11	10	5

1 This age is based on SCRO records up until September 2002

Table B.2 Self-reported offences (detected and undetected)

Type of offence	No. of respondents
Shoplifting	31
Possession of drugs	28
Breach of the Peace	24
Assault	23
Theft	21
Housebreaking	20
Supply of drugs	12
Fraud	12
Motorbike/car theft	10
Serious assault	9
Vandalism	9
Police assault	9
Road Traffic Act offences	9
Reset	8
Under-age drinking	6
Carrying offensive weapon	5
Drunk and disorderly/incapable	4
Resisting arrest	4
Breaking into cars	3
Malicious damage	2
Fighting	2
Attempted murder	2
Grievous bodily harm	2
Trespass	2
Female prostitution	2
Robbery	2
Handling explosives	1
Child neglect	1
Solvent abuse	1
Abduction	1
Indecent exposure	1
Indecent assault	1
Fire-raising	1
Brandishing a gun	1
Armed robbery	1
Mugging	1
Criminal damage	1
Absconding	1
Non-payment of TV licence	1
Wasting police time	1
Racially-aggravated assault	1
Perverting the course of justice	1
Contempt of court	1

The following tables briefly illustrate the range of circumstances of respondents at interview.

Table B.3 Age of respondents

	18–21	22–25	26–29	30–33
Male	9	7	4	–
Female	7	5	7	1
Total	16	12	11	1

As can be seen from Table B.3, the women tended to be older than the men, with eight of the women compared with only three of the men being aged 26 or over. This may partly account for the fact that more women than men said at the time of interview that they had stopped offending.

Table B.4 Housing situation of respondents

	Living with parent(s)	Living with partner	Living alone	Living in a hostel	Homeless
Male	7	7	4	–	2
Female	5	5	8	1	1
Total	12	12	12	1	3

Equal proportions of men and women were living with parents or partners, whilst twice as many women as men were living alone. Seven of the men and 16 of the women had children, and whilst all these women were living with one or more of their children, only those men still with their partners were living with their children.

Table B.5 Age of onset of offending

Age of onset	Male (n=20)	Female (n =20)	Total (n=40)
8–11	6	5	11
12–15	12	9	21
16–19	2	4	6
20–23	0	2	2

Just over a quarter of the sample, with similar numbers of male to female respondents, stated that they had started offending before the age of 12, but there is a greater divergence of the sexes thereafter, with 12 of the young men compared with 9 of the young women saying that they started offending between the ages of 12 and 15. Only 2 young men started after the age of 16, compared with 6 young women.

Table B.6 Average number of previous offences (SCRO data)

	Number of previous offences				
	3–9	10–20	21–40	41–60	61+
Male	–	3	10	4	3
Female	7	6	4	2	1
Total	7	9	14	6	4

The 40 individuals in this sample were above average in terms of type of offence committed and level of persistence. The men had a much higher number of previous offences (calculated from SCRO data) than the women (a total of 765 accruing throughout the men's offending histories up until September 2002, compared with 411 for the women). For those contacted via the voluntary organization providing intensive probation supervision, the average number of previous offences was 38 for the 20 men and 20 for the 7 women. For the remaining 13 young women contacted via social work departments (all of whom had been on probation, albeit not intensive probation), the average number of previous offences was 17.

Table B.7 Most common previous disposals (SCRO data)

	Type of previous disposal				
	Custody	Community Service Orders	Probation (inc. intensive probation[1])	Fines	Admonition
Male	18	15	20	19	17
Female	4	2	20	15	15
Total	22	17	40	34	32

1 SCRO data do not allow a distinction to be drawn between straight probation and intensive probation.

The majority of the men had received custodial sentences and community service orders in the past, thus reflecting their high tariff status as offenders. All of the respondents had been subject to probation orders and all the men had been on intensive probation orders in the past. Half of the female respondents suggested they had been in custody before, mainly on remand but four had also received custodial sentences.

Notes

I INTRODUCTION

1 There tends to be a strong and invariant correlation between crime and age which is commonly referred to as the 'age–crime curve'. Farrall (2002) depicts the age–crime curve for men as rising rapidly from the early teens to a peak at 17–19, and falling steeply at first, then more gradually into the late twenties. For women, however, the curve rises almost as steeply as for men initially, reaches a plateau between 14 and 18, and then declines gradually into the late twenties.

2 The term 'generativity' means, in the context of the desistance literature, the desire to care for others and to feel needed through productive and intergenerational outlets. Maruna (2001) cites a typology of generativity by Stewart *et al.* (1988) which includes caring for others; making a lasting contribution; concern for one's offspring; being needed; and productivity/growth.

3 Whilst 39 of the total sample of 40 fall into the age range 18–30, one female was aged 33.

2 OFFENDING AND DESISTANCE IN THEORY

1 This chapter draws on a more extensive literature review in Barry (2004).

4 STARTING OFFENDING

1 From 1971 in Scotland, the children's hearings system constituted a welfare-based tribunal to deal with child offenders as well as those beyond parental or educational control or in moral or other danger.

6 IN SEARCH OF SOCIAL RECOGNITION

1 Whilst Bourdieu tends to refrain from any discussion of *expenditure* of capital, focusing almost exclusively on the *accumulation* of capital, his analogy with economics is deployed here to describe the uses to which young people can put their capital in the pursuit of mainstream social

integration, namely through taking on responsibility and generativity (see Chapter 3, Table 3.1).

2 Living with one's parents is not, of itself, a reason why an individual may not have responsibilities or stop offending; indeed, Graham and Bowling (1995) suggest that for young men in particular, living at home into their twenties had a positive influence on their likelihood of desisting from offending.

3 Whilst ex-offenders are no doubt 'experts on the subject of deviance and desistance' (Maruna, 2001: 120), there is, nevertheless, resistance to using ex-offenders as counsellors or befrienders in the criminal justice field. Such resistance can come as much from middle-class professionals in the field as from the wider public (Leary, 1962, cited in Maruna, 2001). In the USA as in the UK, prison-based programmes involving inmates 'educating' or 'scaring' children and young people on day visits to the prison have had mixed responses and are inconclusive in the extent to which they either help inmates or the young visitors to change their behaviour or attitudes (Lloyd, 1995). However, Maruna argues that the reforming abilities of involving offenders in rehabilitation schemes are significant and such generativity acts as an alternative source of 'empowerment and potency' to offending behaviour (2002: 121).

APPENDIX A: METHODOLOGY

1 Cameron and Telfer (2004) note that most group-work programmes are male-oriented but that young women have specific problems in relation to their offending behaviour which require customized programmes. Covington (1998) also suggests that women offenders require women-only programmes in order to address their particular criminogenic needs.

2 All bar one man, in prison at the time of the interview, agreed to the interview being taped. However, permission to tape an interview was refused by prison staff for a further young man in custody.

3 It should be pointed out that I did not offer, and none requested, payment for their time during the course of this research. Not only did they give of their time without expectation of payment, they were also all happy for me to contact them again should I require any further information at a later date.

4 Interviews 6, 32 and 33 were not used for the purposes of this research study because the respondents did not meet the criteria for eligibility, namely 2+ previous convictions.

5 'Triangulation' (Denzin, 1970) to a certain extent resolves the issue of competing perceptions or realities from different empirical sources, in that the researcher can gain the same information from several different sources in order to estimate its accuracy.

6 'Zero sum', according to Scott (2001: 6–7), means that 'power relations are seen as asymmetrical, hierarchical relations ... in which one agent can gain only at the expense of another ... there is a given distribution of power ... [involving] both winners and losers.' 'Non-zero sum', on the other hand, suggests that there is an infinite quantity of power, in which there are only winners.

References

Adler, P. (1985) 'Wheeling and dealing: an ethnography of upper-level drug dealing and smuggling community', in S. Farrall (2000) (ed.) *The Termination of Criminal Careers*, Aldershot: Ashgate.

Agnew, R. (1992) 'Foundation for a general strain theory of crime and delinquency', *Criminology*, Vol. 30, No. 1: 47–87.

Allatt, P. and Yeandle, S. (1992) *Youth Unemployment and the Family: Voices Of Disordered Times*, London: Routledge.

Archard, D. (1993) *Children: Rights and Childhood*, London: Routledge.

Aries, P. (1962) *Centuries of Childhood*, London: Jonathan Cape.

Barnardo's (1996) *Young People's Social Attitudes: Having Their Say – The Views of 12–19 Year Olds*, Ilford: Barnardo's.

Barry, M. (2000) 'The mentor/monitor debate in criminal justice: "what works" for offenders', *British Journal of Social Work*, Vol. 30: 575–95.

Barry, M. (2001a) *A Sense of Purpose: Care Leavers' Views and Experiences of Growing Up*, London: Save the Children/Joseph Rowntree Foundation.

Barry, M. (2001b) *Challenging Transitions: Young People's Views and Experiences of Growing Up*, London: Save the Children/Joseph Rowntree Foundation.

Barry, M. (2002) 'Minor rights and major concerns: the views of young people in care', in B. Franklin (ed.) *The New Handbook of Children's Rights: Comparative Policy and Practice*, London: Routledge.

Barry, M. (2004) *Understanding Youth Offending: In Search of 'Social Recognition'*, unpublished PhD thesis, Stirling: University of Stirling.

Barry, M. (2005) 'Introduction', in M. Barry (ed.) *Youth Policy and Social Inclusion: Critical Debates with Young People*, London: Routledge.

Bates, I. and Riseborough, G. (1993) *Youth and Inequality*, Buckingham: Open University Press.

Beck, U. (1992) *Risk Society: Towards a New Modernity*, London: Sage.

Becker, H. (1963) *Outsiders: Studies in the Sociology of Deviance*, New York: Free Press.

Blumstein, A. and Cohen, J. (1987) 'Characterizing criminal careers', *Science*, Vol. 237: 985–91.

Blumstein, A., Cohen, J. and Farrington, D.P. (1988) 'Criminal career research: its value for criminology', *Criminology*, Vol. 26, No. 1: 1–35.

Bottoms, A. (1993) 'Recent criminological and social theory', in D. Farrington, R. Sampson and P. Wilkstrom (eds) *Integrating Individual and Ecological Aspects of Crime*, Stockholm: National Council for Crime Prevention.

Bottoms, A. and Wiles, P. (1992) 'Explanations of crime and place', in D.J. Evans, N.R. Fyfe and D.T. Herbert (eds) *Crime, Policing and Place*, London: Routledge.

Bottoms, A., Shapland, J., Costello, A., Holmes, D. and Grant, M. (2004) 'Towards desistance: theoretical underpinnings for an empirical study', *The Howard Journal*, Vol. 43, No. 4: 368–89.

Bourdieu, P. (1977) *Outline of a Theory of Practice*, Cambridge: Cambridge University Press.

Bourdieu, P. (1984) *Distinction: A Social Critique of the Judgement of Taste'* (trans. Richard Nice), London: Routledge.

Bourdieu, P. (1986) 'The forms of capital', in J.G. Richardson (ed.) *Handbook of Theory and Research for the Sociology of Education*, Westport, CT: Greenwood Press.

Bourdieu, P. (1989) 'Social space and symbolic power', *Sociological Theory*, Vol. 7: 14–25.

Bourdieu, P. (1990) *In Other Words: Essays Towards a Reflexive Sociology* (trans.M. Adamson), Cambridge: Polity Press.

Bourdieu, P (1991) *Language and Symbolic Power*, edited and introduced by J.B. Thompson, (trans G. Raymond and M. Adamson), Cambridge: Polity Press.

Bourdieu, P. (1997) 'The forms of capital', in A.H. Halsey, H. Lauder, P. Brown and A. Stuart Wells (eds) *Education: Culture, Economy, Society*, Oxford: Oxford University Press.

Bourdieu, P. (1998) *Practical Reason*, Cambridge: Polity Press.

Bourdieu, P. and Wacquant, L. (1992) *An Invitation to Reflexive Sociology*, Cambridge: Polity Press.

Braithwaite, J. (1989) *Crime, Shame and Reintegration*, Cambridge: Cambridge University Press.

Brake, M. (1985) *Comparative Youth Culture*, London: Routledge and Kegan Paul.

Bright, J. (1996) 'Preventing youth crime in high crime areas', in S. Asquith (ed.) *Children and Young People in Conflict with the Law*, London: Jessica Kingsley.

British Sociological Association (1996) *Guidance Notes: Statement of Ethical Practice*, Durham: BSA.

Bromley, D. (1993) *Reputation, Image and Impression Management*, Chichester: Wiley.

Brown, S. (1998) *Understanding Youth and Crime: Listening to Youth?*, Buckingham: Open University Press.

Bryman, A. (1988) *Quantity and Quality in Social Research*, London: Unwin Hyman.

Buckle, A. and Farrington, D. (1984) 'An observational study of shoplifting', *British Journal of Criminology*, Vol. 24 No. 1: 63–73.

Burnett, R. (2003) 'To re-offend or not to re-offend? The ambivalence of convicted property offenders', in S. Maruna and R. Immarigeon (eds) *After Crime and Punishment: Ex-Offender Reintegration and Desistance from Crime*, Albany, NY: SUNY Press.

Butters, S. (1976) 'The logic-of-enquiry of participant observation', in S. Hall and T. Jefferson (eds) *Resistance Through Rituals*, London: Hutchinson and Co.

Bynner, J., Chisholm, L. and Furlong, A. (eds) (1997) *Youth, Citizenship and Social Change in a European Context*, Aldershot: Ashgate.

Callinicos, A. (1999) 'Social theory put to the test of politics: Pierre Bourdieu and Anthony Giddens', *New Left Review*, Vol. 236: 77–102.

Cameron, H. and Telfer, J. (2004) 'Cognitive-behavioural group work: its application to specific offender groups', *Howard Journal*, Vol. 43, No. 1: 47–64.

Campbell, A. (1981) *Girl Delinquents*, Oxford: Blackwell.

Chesney-Lind, M. (1997) *The Female Offender: Girls, Women and Crime*, Thousand Oaks, CA: Sage.

Chisholm, L. (1993) 'Youth transitions in Britain on the threshold of a "New Europe"', *Journal of Education Policy*, Vol. 8, No. 1: 29–41.

Cloward, R. and Ohlin, L. (1961) *Delinquency and Opportunity: A Theory of Delinquent Gangs*, London: Routledge and Kegan Paul.

Coffield, F., Borrill, C. and Marshall, S. (1986) *Growing Up at the Margins*, Milton Keynes: Open University Press.

Cohen, A. (1955) *Delinquent Boys: The Culture of the Gang*, London: Free Press.

Cohen, P. and Ainley, P. (2000) 'In the country of the blind? Youth studies and cultural studies in Britain', *Journal of Youth Studies*, Vol. 3, No. 1: 79–95.

Coleman, J.S. (1988) 'Social capital in the creation of human capital', *American Journal of Sociology*, Vol. 94, Supplement: S95–S120.

Coles, B. (1995) *Youth and Social Policy: Youth Citizenship and Young Careers*, London, UCL Press.

Coles, B. (2000) *Joined-up Youth Research, Policy and Practice: A New Agenda for Change?*, Leicester: Youth Work Press.

Cornish, D. and Clarke, R.V. (1986) *The Reasoning Criminal*, New York: Springer-Verlag.

Cote, J. (2002) 'The role of identity capital in the transition to adulthood: the individualization thesis examined', *Journal of Youth Studies*, Vol. 5, No. 2: 117–34.

Covington, J. (1985) 'Gender differences in criminality among heroin users', *Journal of Research in Crime and Delinquency*, Vol. 22, No. 4: 329–54.

Covington, S. (1998) 'The relational theory of women's psychological development: implications for the criminal justice system', in R.T. Zaplin (ed.) *Female Offenders: Critical Perspectives and Effective Interventions*, Gaithersburg, MD: Aspen Publishers Inc.

Craib, I. (1992) *Modern Social Theory: From Parsons to Habermas* (2nd edition), Hemel Hempstead: Harvester Wheatsheaf.

Craine, S. (1997) 'The "Black Magic Roundabout": cyclical transitions, social exclusion and alternative careers', in R. MacDonald (ed.) *Youth, the 'Underclass' and Social Exclusion*, London: Routledge.

Cunneen, C. and White, R. (2002) *Juvenile Justice: Youth and Crime in Australia*, Oxford: Oxford University Press.

Cusson, M. and Pinsonneault, P. (1986) 'The decision to give up crime', in D. Cornish and R.V. Clarke (eds) *The Reasoning Criminal*, New York: Springer-Verlag.

Davies, N. (2003a) 'The war on crime: at the frontline', *The Guardian*, 10 July.

Davies, N. (2003b) 'Unreliable sources: exploding the myth of the falling crime rate', *The Guardian*, 10 July.

Dearden, C. and Becker, S. (2000) *Growing Up Caring: Vulnerability and Transition to Adulthood – Young Carers' Experiences*, Leicester: Youth Work Press/Joseph Rowntree Foundation.

Denzin, N.K. (1970) *The Research Act*, Chicago, IL: Aldine.

de Vries, E. (1968) 'Explorations into Reciprocity', in E. de Vries (ed.) *Essays on Reciprocity*, The Hague: Mouton.

Downes, D. (1966) *The Delinquent Solution*, London: Routledge and Kegan Paul.

Downes, D. and Rock, P. (1988) *Understanding Deviance: A Guide to the Sociology of Crime and Rule Breaking* (2nd edition), Oxford: Clarendon Press.

Eley, S., Gallop, K., McIvor, G., Morgan, K. and Yates, R. (2002) *Drug Treatment and Testing Orders: Evaluation of the Scottish Pilots*, Edinburgh: The Stationery Office.

Emler, N. (1990) 'A social psychology of reputation', in W. Stroebe and M. Hewstone (eds) *European Review of Social Psychology, Volume 1*, Chichester: John Wiley & Sons.

Emler, N. and Reicher, S. (1995) *Adolescence and Delinquency: The Collective Management of Reputation*, Oxford: Blackwell.

Emler, N., Reicher, S. and Ross, A. (1987) 'The social context of delinquent conduct', *Journal of Child Psychology and Psychiatry*, Vol. 28, No. 1: 99–109.

Emond, R. (2000) 'Survival of the skilful: an ethnographic study of two groups of young people in residential care', unpublished PhD Thesis: Stirling, University of Stirling.

Emsley, C. (1994) 'The history of crime and crime control institutions, c.1770–c.1945', in M. Maguire, R. Morgan and R. Reiner (eds) *The Oxford Handbook of Criminology*, Oxford: Oxford University Press.

Erikson, E. H. (1968) *Identity, Youth and Crisis*, London: Faber and Faber.

Farrall, S. (ed.) (2000) *The Termination of Criminal Careers*, Aldershot: Ashgate.

Farrall, S. (2002) *Rethinking What Works with Offenders*, Cullompton, Devon: Willan.

Farrall, S. and Bowling, B. (1997) 'Structuration, Human Development and Desistance from Crime', paper presented to the British Criminology Conference, Belfast, July.

Farrall, S. and Bowling, B. (1999) 'Structuration, human development and desistance from crime', *British Journal of Criminology*, Vol. 39, No. 2: 253–68.

Farrington, D. (1986) 'Stepping stones to adult criminal careers', in D. Olweus, J. Blackand and M. R. Yarrow (eds) *Development of Antisocial and Prosocial Behaviour*, New York: Academic Press.

Farrington, D. (1995) The Twelfth Jack Tizard Memorial Lecture: The development of offending and antisocial behaviour from childhood: key findings from the Cambridge Study in Delinquent Development, *Journal of Child Psychology and Psychiatry*, Vol. 36: 929–64.

Farrington, D. (1997) 'Human Development and Criminal Careers', in M. Maguire, R. Morgan and R. Reiner (eds) (2nd edition) *The Oxford Handbook of Criminology*, Oxford: Oxford University Press.

Farrington, D. and Hawkins, J. (1991) 'Predicting participation, early onset and later persistence in officially recorded offending', *Criminal Behaviour and Mental Health*, Vol. 1: 1–33.

Farrington, D., Gallagher, B., Morley, L., St. Ledger, R. and West, D.J. (1986) 'Unemployment, school leaving, and crime', *British Journal of Criminology*, Vol. 26, No. 4: 335–56.

Fenwick, M. and Hayward, K. (2000) 'Cultural criminology', in J. Pickford (ed.) *Youth Justice: Theory and Practice*, London: Cavendish.

Ferrell, J. (1993) *Crimes of Style: Urban Graffiti and the Politics of Criminality*, New York: Garland.

Ferrell, J. (1995) 'Style matters: criminal identity and social control', in J. Ferrell and C. Sanders (eds) *Cultural Criminology*, Boston, MA: Northeastern University Press.

Ferrell, J. and Sanders C. (eds) (1995) *Cultural Criminology*, Boston, MA: Northeastern University Press.

Flood-Page, C., Campbell, S., Harrington, V. and Miller, J. (2000) *Youth Crime: Findings from the 1998/99 Youth Lifestyles Survey*, Home Office Research Study 209, London: Home Office.

Fowler, B. (ed.) (2000) *Reading Bourdieu on Society and Culture*, Oxford: Blackwell.

Franklin, B. (ed.) (2002) *The New Handbook of Children's Rights: Comparative Policy and Practice*, London: Routledge.

Fukuyama, F. (1995) *Trust: The Social Virtues and the Creation of Prosperity*, London: Hamish Hamilton.

Furlong, A. and Cartmel, F. (1997) *Young People and Social Change: Individualization and Risk in Late Modernity*, Milton Keynes: Open University Press.

Gelsthorpe, L. and Morris, A. (Eds) (1990) 'Introduction: transforming and transgressing criminology', *Feminist Perspectives in Criminology*, Buckingham: Open University Press.

Giddens, A. (1976) *New Rules of Sociological Method*, London: Hutchinson.

Giddens, A. (1979) *Central Problems in Social Theory: Action, Structure and Contradiction in Social Analysis*, London: Macmillan.

Giddens, A. (1984) *The Constitution of Society*, Cambridge: Polity Press.

Giddens, A. (1991) 'Structuration theory: past, present and future', in C. Bryant and D. Jary (eds) *Giddens' Theory of Structuration: A Critical Appreciation*, London: Routledge.

Gillies, V., Holland, J. and Ribbens McCarthy, J. (2002) 'Past/present/future: time and the meaning of change in the "family"', in G. Allan and G. Jones (eds) *Social Relations and the Life Course*, Basingstoke: Palgrave.

Gilligan, C. (1982) *In A Different Voice: Psychological Theory and Women's Development*, Cambridge, MA: Harvard University Press.

Glaser, D. (1980) 'The interplay of theory, issues, policy and data', in M. Klein and K. Tielmann (eds) *Handbook of Criminal Justice Evaluation*, Beverley Hills, CA: Sage.

Glueck, S. and Glueck, E. (1940) *Unraveling Juvenile Delinquency*, New York: Commonwealth Fund.

Gottfredson, M. and Hirschi, T. (1990) *A General Theory of Crime*, Stanford, CA: Stanford University Press.

Graham, J. and Bowling, B. (1995) *Young People and Crime*, London: Home Office.

Greenberg, D. (1979) 'Delinquency and the age structure of society', in S. Messinger and E. Bittner (eds) *Criminology Review Yearbook*, Beverly Hills, CA: Sage.

Hall, S. and Jefferson, T. (1976) *Resistance Through Rituals*, London: Hutchinson and Co.

Harnett, R., Thom, B., Herring, R. and Kelly, M. (2000) 'Alcohol in transition: towards a model of young men's drinking styles', *Journal of Youth Studies*, Vol. 3, No. 1: 61–77.

Haugaard, M. (ed.) (2002) *Power: A Reader*, Manchester: Manchester University Press.

Heidensohn, F. (1985) *Women and Crime*, London: Macmillan.

Heidensohn, F. (1994) 'Gender and crime', in M. Maguire, R. Morgan and R. Reiner (eds) *The Oxford Handbook of Criminology*, Oxford: Oxford University Press.

Heidensohn, F. (1996) *Women and Crime* (2nd edition), London: Macmillan.

Holland, J., Gillies, V. and McCarthy, J.R. (1999) 'Living on the Edge: Accounts of Young People Leaving Childhood Behind', paper presented to the ESA Conference, Amsterdam, August.

Holroyd, R. (2002) '"Standing Out" and "Fitting in": Negotiating the Complexities of Peer Culture in Adolescence', paper presented to the Young People 2002 Conference, Keele University.

James, A. and Prout, A. (1997) 'Re-presenting childhood', in A. James and A. Prout (eds) *Constructing and Reconstructing Childhood*, London: Falmer Press.

Jamieson, J., McIvor, G. and Murray, C. (1999) *Understanding Offending Among Young People*, Edinburgh: The Stationery Office.

Jeffs, T. and Smith, M. (1998) 'The problem of "youth" for youth work', *Youth and Policy*, No. 62: 45–66.

Jenkins, D. (1992) *Pierre Bourdieu*, London: Routledge.

Jones, G. (1995) *Leaving Home*, Buckingham: Open University Press.

Jones, G. (1996) 'Deferred citizenship: a coherent policy of exclusion?', *Young People Now*, 26 March: 26–7.

Jones, G. and Wallace, C. (1992) *Youth, Family and Citizenship*, Milton Keynes: Open University Press.

Jones, S. (1985) 'The analysis of depth interviews', in R. Walker (ed.) *Applied Qualitative Research*, Aldershot: Gower.

Kandel, D.B. (1978) 'Homophily, selection and socialization in adolescent friendships', *American Journal of Sociology*, Vol. 84: 427–36.

Katz, J. (1988) *Seductions of Crime: Moral and Sensual Attraction in Doing Evil*, New York: Basic Books.

Katz, J. (1991) 'The motivation of persistent robbers', in M. Tonry (ed.) *Crime and Justice: An Annual Review of Research*, Vol. 14, Chicago, IL: Chicago University Press.

Katz, R. (2000) 'Explaining girls' and women's crime and desistance in the context of their victimization experiences', *Violence Against Women*, Vol. 6, No. 6: 633–60.

Kearns, A. and Parkinson, M. (2001) 'The significance of neighbourhood', *Urban Studies*, Vol. 38, No. 12: 2103–10.

Knight, B.J. and West, D.J. (1975) 'Temporary and continuing delinquency', *British Journal of Criminology*, Vol. 15, No. 1, pp. 43–50.

Laub, J. and Sampson, R. (2003) *Shared Beginnings, Divergent Lives: Delinquent Boys to Age 70*, Cambridge, MA: Harvard University Press.

Laub, J., Nagin, D. and Sampson, R. (1998) 'Trajectories of change in criminal offending: good marriages and the desistance process', *American Sociological Review*, Vol. 63: 225–38.

LeBlanc, M. and Frechette, M. (1989) *Male Criminal Activity from Childhood through Youth*, New York: Springer-Verlag.

Leibrich, J. (1992) *Methdology for a Study on Desistance from Crime: A Working Paper*, Wellington: Department of Justice.

Leibrich, J. (1993) *Straight to the Point: Angles on Giving Up Crime*, Dunedin, New Zealand: University of Otago Press.

Lister, R., Middleton, S., Smith, N., Vincent, J. and Cox, L. (2002) *Negotiating Transitions to Citizenship*, http://www.regard.ac.uk.

Lloyd, C. (1995) *To Scare Straight or Educate? The British Experience of Day Visits to Prison for Young People*, Home Office Research Study 149, London: Home Office.

Loeber, R., Southamer-Loeber, M., Van Kammen, W. and Farrington, D.P. (1991) 'Initiation, escalation and desistance in juvenile offending and their correlates', *Journal of Criminal Law and Criminology*, Vol. 82: 36–82.

MacDonald, R. (1997) 'Youth, social exclusion and the millennium', in R. MacDonald (ed.) *Youth, The 'Underclass' and Social Exclusion*, London: Routledge.

MacDonald, R. and Marsh, J. (2005) *Disconnected Youth? Growing up in Britain's Poor Neighbourhoods*, Basingstoke: Palgrave Macmillan.

MacDonald, R., Mason, P., Shildrick, T., Webster, C. Johnston, L. and Ridley, L. (2001) 'Snakes and ladders: in defence of studies of youth transition', *Sociological Research Online*, Vol. 5, No. 4, http://www.socresonline.org.uk/5/4/macdonald.html.

McIvor, G. (1992) *Sentenced To Serve: The Operation and Impact of Community Service by Offenders*, Aldershot: Avebury.

McIvor, G. and Barry, M. (1998a) *Social Work and Criminal Justice: Probation*, Edinburgh: The Stationery Office.

McIvor, G. and Barry, M. (1998b) *Social Work and Criminal Justice: Throughcare*, Edinburgh: The Stationery Office.

McIvor, G., Murray, C. and Jamieson, J. (2004) 'Is desistance from crime different for girls?', in S. Maruna and R. Immarigeon (eds) *After Crime and Punishment: Ex-Offender Reintegration and Desistance from Crime*, Albany, NY: SUNY Press.

MacRae, R. (2002) 'Becoming a clubber: transitions, identities and lifestyles', unpublished PhD thesis, Stirling: University of Stirling.

McRobbie, A. (2000) *Feminism and Youth Culture* (2nd edition), Basingstoke: Macmillan.

Maruna, S. (1998) *Redeeming One's Self: How Reformed Ex-Offenders Make Sense of Their Lives*, unpublished doctoral dissertation, Evanston: IL: Northwestern University.

Maruna, S. (2001) *Making Good: How Ex-Convicts Reform and Rebuild Their Lives*, Washington DC: American Psychological Association.

Matsueda, R. and Heimer, K. (1997) 'A symbolic interactionist theory of role-transitions, role-commitments, and delinquency', in T.P. Thornberry (ed.) *Developmental Theories of Crime and Delinquency*, New Brunswick, NJ: Transaction Publishers.

Matza, D. (1964) *Delinquency and Drift*, New York: Wiley.

Matza, D. (1969) *Becoming Deviant*, Englewood Cliffs, NJ: Prentice-Hall.

May, T. (1996) *Situating Social Theory*, Buckingham: Open University Press.

Merton, R. (1957) *Social Theory and Social Structure*, New York: Free Press.

Messerschmidt, J.W. (1995) 'From patriarchy to gender: feminist theory, criminology and the challenge of diversity', in N. Rafter and F. Heidensohn (eds) *International Feminist Perspectives in Criminology: Engendering a Discipline*, Buckingham: Open University Press.

Miles, S. (2000) *Youth Lifestyles in a Changing World*, Buckingham: Open University Press.

Miles, S., Cliff, D. and Burr, V. (1998) '"Fitting in and sticking out": consumption, consumer meanings and the construction of young people's identities', *Journal of Youth Studies*, Vol. 1, No. 1: 81–96.

Miller, W.B. (1958) 'Lower class culture as a generating milieu of gang delinquency', *Journal of Social Issues*, No. 14: 5–19.

Moffitt, T.E. (1993) 'Adolescence-limited and life-course-persistent antisocial behaviour: a developmental taxonomy', *Psychological Review*, Vol. 100: 674–701.

Moffitt, T.E. (1997) 'Adolescence-limited and life-course persistent offending: a complementary pair of developmental theories', in T.P. Thornberry (ed.) *Developmental Theories of Crime and Delinquency*, New Brunswick: Transaction Publishers.

Morris, A. (1987) *Women, Crime and Criminal Justice*, Oxford: Basil Blackwell.

Morrow, V. (1999) 'Conceptualising social capital in relation to the well-being of children and young people: a critical review', *The Sociological Review*, Vol. 47: 744–65.

Morrow, V. (2001) 'Young people's explanations and experiences of social exclusion: retrieving Bourdieu's concept of social capital', *International Journal of Sociology and Social Policy*, Vol. 21, No. 4/5/6: 37–63.

Muncie, J. (1999) *Youth and Crime: A Critical Introduction*, London: Sage.

Mungham, G. (1982) 'Workless youth as a moral panic', in T. Rees and P. Atkinson (eds) *Youth Unemployment and State Intervention*, London: Routledge and Kegan Paul.

Musgrove, F. (1964) *Youth and the Social Order*, London: Routledge and Kegan Paul.

Oakley, A. (1981) 'Interviewing women: a contradiction in terms', in H. Roberts (ed.) *Doing Feminist Research*, London: Routledge and Kegan Paul.

Parker, J. G. and Asher, R.S. (1987) 'Peer relations and later personal adjustment: are low-accepted children at risk?', *Psychological Bulletin*, Vol. 102: 357–89.

Phoenix, A. (1994) 'Practising feminist research: the intersection of gender and race in the research process', in M. Maynard and J. Purvis (eds) *Researching Women's Lives from a Feminist Perspective*, London: Taylor and Francis.

Portes, A. and Landolt, P. (1996) 'The downside of social capital', *The American Prospect*, No. 26: 18–21.

Prasad, R. (2003) 'A leap of faith', *The Guardian*, 16 July.

Pudney, S. (2002) *The Road to Ruin? Sequences of Initiation Into Drug Use and Offending by Young People in Britain*, Home Office Research Study 253, London: Home Office.

Putnam, R.D. (1993) *Making Democracy Work: Civic Traditions in Modern Italy*, Princeton NJ: Princeton University Press.

Putnam, R.D. (2000) *Bowling Alone: The Collapse and Revival of American Community*, New York: Simon and Schuster.

Raffo, C. and Reeves, M. (2000) 'Youth transitions and social exclusion: developments in social capital theory', *Journal of Youth Studies*, Vol. 3, No. 2: 147–66.

Reiss, A.J. (1988) 'Co-offending and criminal careers', in M. Tonry and N. Morris (eds) *Crime and Justice: A Review of Research* Vol. 10, Chicago, IL: University of Chicago Press.

Roberts, K. (2003) 'Problems and priorities for the sociology of youth', in A. Bennett, M. Cieslik and S. Miles (eds) *Researching Youth*, Basingstoke: Palgrave Macmillan.

Rolfe, A. (2005) '"There's helping and there's hindering": young mothers, support and control', in M. Barry (ed.) *Youth Policy and Social Inclusion: Critical Debates With Young People*, London: Routledge.

Rowe, D.C., Wouldbroun, E.J. and Gulley, B.L. (1994) 'Peers and friends as nonshared environmental influences', in E.M. Hetherington, D. Reiss and R. Plomin (eds), *Separate Social Worlds of Siblings*, Hillsdale, NJ: Erlbaum.

Rudd, P. and Evans, K. (1998) 'Structure and agency in youth transitions: student experiences of vocational further education', *Journal of Youth Studies*, Vol. 1, No. 1: 39–62.

Rutherford, A. (1986) *Growing Out of Crime: The New Era*, Winchester: Waterside Press.

Rutter, M. (1996) 'Transitions and turning points in developmental psychopathology: as applied to the age span between childhood and mid-adulthood', *International Journal of Behavioural Development*, Vol. 19: 603–26.

Rutter, M., Giller, H. and Hagell, A. (1998) *Antisocial Behaviour by Young People*, Cambridge: Cambridge University Press.

Sampson, R.J. and Laub, J.H. (1993) *Crime in the Making: Pathways and Turning Points Through Life*, Cambridge, MA: Harvard University Press.

Scott, J. (2001) *Power*, Cambridge: Polity Press.

Scottish Executive (2002) *Criminal Proceedings in Scottish Courts, 2001*, Statistical Bulletin, Criminal Justice Series, Edinburgh: Scottish Executive.

Scottish Office (1998) *Women Offenders – A Safer Way*, A Review of Community Disposals and the Use of Custody for Women Offenders in Scotland, Edinburgh: The Stationery Office.

Scraton, P. (1990) 'Scientific knowledge or masculine discourses?', in L. Gelsthorpe and A. Morris (eds) *Feminist Perspectives in Criminology*, Buckingham: Open University Press.

Sennett, R. (2003) *Respect: The Formation of Character in a World of Inequality*, London: Allen Lane.

Sennett, R. and Cobb, J. (1972) *The Hidden Injuries of Class*, Cambridge: Cambridge University Press.

Shover, N. (1996) *Great Pretenders: Pursuits and Careers of Persistent Thieves*, Boulder, CO: Westview Press.

Shover, N. and Thompson, C. (1992) 'Age, differential expectations, and crime desistance', *Criminology*, Vol. 30, No. 1: 89–104.

Skeggs, B. (1997) *Formations of Class and Gender: Becoming Respectable*, London: Sage.

Smith, D. (1986) *Crime, Space and Society*, Cambridge: Cambridge University Press.

Sommers, I., Baskin, D. and Fagan, J. (1994) 'Getting out of the life: crime desistance by female street offenders', *Deviant Behaviour: An Interdisciplinary Journal*, Vol. 15: 125–49.

Stephen, D. (2000) 'Young women construct themselves: social identity, self-concept and psychosocial well-being in homeless facilities', *Journal of Youth Studies*, Vol. 3, No. 4: 445–60.

Stephen, D. and Squires, P. (2003) '"Adults don't realise how sheltered they are": a contribution to the debate on youth transitions from some voices on the margins', *Journal of Youth Studies*, Vol. 6, No. 2, June: 145–64.

Stewart, A.J., Franz, C. and Layton, L. (1988) 'The changing self: using personal documents to study lives', *Journal of Personality*, Vol. 56: 41–74.

Stewart, J., Smith, D. and Stewart, G. (1994) *Understanding Offending Behaviour*, Harlow: Longman.

Sutherland, E.H. and Cressey, D.R. (1970) *Criminology* (8th edition), Philadelphia, PA: Lippincott.

Sutherland, E.H. and Cressey, D.R. (1978) *Criminology* (10th edition), Philadelphia, PA: Lippincott.

Sykes, G.M. and Matza, D. (1957) 'Techniques of neutralization: a theory of delinquency', *American Sociological Review*, Vol. 22: 664–70.

Taylor, A. (1993) *Women Drug Users: An Ethnography of a Female Injecting Community*, Oxford: Clarendon Press.

Taylor, D. (2000) 'The word on the street: advertising, youth culture and legitimate speech in drug education', *Journal of Youth Studies*, Vol. 3, No. 3: 333–52.

Thomson, R. and Holland, J. (2002) *Inventing Adulthood: Young People's Strategies for Transition*, Swindon: ESRC.

Thomson, R., Henderson, S. and Holland, J. (2003) 'Making the most of what you've got? resources, values and inequalities in young women's transitions to adulthood', *Educational Review*, Vol. 55, No. 1: 33–46.

Thornberry, T.P. (1997) 'Introduction: some advantages of developmental and life-course perspectives for the study of crime and delinquency', in T.P. Thornberry (ed.), *Developmental Theories of Crime and Delinquency*, New Brunswick, NJ: Transaction Publishers.

Thornberry, T.P. and Krohn, M.D. (1997) 'Peers, drug use and delinquency', in D. Stoff, J. Breiling and J.D. Maser (eds), *Handbook of Antisocial Behaviour*, New York: Wiley.

Thornberry, T.P., Lizotte, A., Krohn, M., Farnworth, M. and Joon Jang, S. (1991) 'Testing interactional theory: an examination of reciprocal causal relationships among family, school and delinquency', *Journal of Criminal Law and Criminology*, Vol. 82: 3–35.

Turner, V. (1967) *The Forest of Symbols: Aspects of Ndombu Ritual*, Ithaca, NY: Cornell University Press.

Turner, V. (1969) *The Ritual Process: Structure and Anti-Structure*, Chicago: Aldine.

Ungar, M. (2000) 'The myth of peer pressure', *Adolescence*, Vol. 35, No. 137, Spring: 167–80.

Utting, D., Bright, J. and Henricson, C. (1993) *Crime and the Family: Improving Child-Rearing and Preventing Delinquency*, London: Family Policy Studies Centre.

Waiton, S. (2001) 'Adult Regulation of Adolescent Peer Relations', paper presented at the Strathclyde Youth Conference, Glasgow.

Wallace, C. (1987) *For Richer, for Poorer: Growing Up In and Out of Work*, London: Tavistock.

Warr, M. and Stafford, M. (1991) 'The influence of delinquent peers', *Criminology*, Vol. 29: 851–65.

Webster, C., Simpson, D., MacDonald, R., Abbas, A., Cieslik, M., Shildrick, T. and Simpson, M. (2004) *Poor Transitions: Social Exclusion and Young Adults*, Bristol: Policy Press.

Willis, P. (1977) *Learning to Labour*, London: Saxon House.

Willis, P. (1990) *Common Culture*, Milton Keynes: Open University Press.

Wilson, J.Q. (1975) *Thinking About Crime*, New York: Vintage.

Wyn, J. and White, R. (1997) *Rethinking Youth*, London: Sage.

Young, J. (1999) *The Exclusive Society*, London: Sage.

Index

Printed in the United States
by Baker & Taylor Publisher Services